One Year Wellness Journey

by

TONI WILLIAMS

While every precaution has been taken in the preparation of this book, the publisher assumes no responsibility for errors or omissions, or for damages resulting from the use of the information contained herein.

ONE YEAR WELLNESS JOURNEY

First edition. October 15, 2024.

Written by Toni Williams.

Table of Contents

One Year Wellness Journey

The Family Well-Being Edition

ONE YEAR WELLNESS JOURNEY BY TONI WILLIAMS

This book is a work of nonfiction.

Any resemblance to persons living or dead, or places, events or locales Is purely memories, experience, and research.

The moments of the author's life and are used inspirationally to encourage positive change.

This book is a collection of health information.

Disclaimer:

As an author and content creator, it is important to clarify that I am not a licensed medical professional, doctor, or therapist. Any information provided in my writing or content is for informational purposes only and should not be considered a substitute for professional medical advice, diagnosis, or treatment.

I strive to provide accurate and up-to-date information based on research and personal experience, but I cannot guarantee the accuracy, completeness, or reliability of the content. It is always recommended to consult with a qualified healthcare professional for any health-related concerns or issues.

I do not assume any responsibility for any individual's use of the information provided, and I disclaim any liability for any loss, injury, or damage resulting from the use of the content on this platform. Readers are encouraged to seek advice and guidance from appropriate medical professionals for personalized healthcare recommendations.

Remember, your health and well-being are important, and it is always best to seek professional medical advice from a qualified healthcare provider.

Honorary Mention

I would like to take the time to acknowledge C. Christopher, and those who were my resources, who provided technical assistance or their knowledge of the subject matter.

Thank you!

Dedication

To all those who have embarked on their own wellness journeys,

May this book serve as a guiding light, inspiring you to take charge of your well-being and embrace a life filled with health, happiness, and fulfillment. May it empower you to overcome challenges, develop resilience, and cultivate a deep sense of self-love and self-care. This book is dedicated to your journey towards holistic wellness, with the hope that it brings you closer to a life of balance, joy, and inner peace.

Acknowledgment:

I would like to express my deepest gratitude to all those who have supported and influenced me throughout the creation of this book. Your unwavering support, encouragement, and belief in my writing have been invaluable.

First and foremost, I am grateful to my family for their love, understanding, and patience during the writing process. Your continual support and belief in my abilities have fueled my inspiration and kept me going through the challenges. K. Smith, E. Williams, S. Christopher, M. Williams, and J. Smith D. Christopher Thank you, you supported and encouraged me during the process.

I extend my heartfelt appreciation to my friends who have been there for me every step of the way. Your presence, conversations, and shared experiences have shaped my perspective on wellness and provided valuable insights that I have incorporated into this book. A. Marks, J. Graham and many more.

I am indebted to my mentor, whose guidance, wisdom, and expertise have been instrumental in guiding me through the writing journey.

Your constructive feedback and unwavering belief in my ideas have been a constant source of inspiration.

I would like to acknowledge the countless authors, researchers, and experts whose work I have drawn upon to create this book. Your valuable contributions to the field of wellness have laid the foundation for my understanding and inspired me to share this knowledge.

Last but certainly not least, I want to express my sincere gratitude to the readers who have chosen to embark on this wellness journey with me. It is for you that this book was written, and it is my hope that it brings you the guidance, motivation, and inspiration needed to create a life of wellness, fulfillment, and joy.

Special Thanks:

A special thanks goes out to the following individuals and organizations, without whom this book would not have been possible:

- Sunny Giovanni: For their generosity in providing resources and research for this book.

- Dr. Jean Akpan: For their valuable insights and expertise in a specific area of wellness.

Your contributions and support have enriched this book and made it a reality. Thank you for being a part of this journey and for your invaluable contributions to the world of wellness.

Embarking on a year-long wellness journey as a family is an exciting and empowering decision. Together, you are committing to prioritizing your physical, mental, and emotional well-being. You will support each other through challenges, celebrate your victories, and create lasting healthy habits that will benefit us for a lifetime.

With motivation as the driving force, you can be determined to make positive changes in the lives of the family. Focus on nourishing your bodies with nutritious food, staying active, practicing mindfulness, and fostering strong connections with each other. This journey is not just about bettering ourselves individually, but also strengthening our bond as a family.

As you take this first step towards a healthier and happier lifestyle, remember that your collective determination and support will be the key to success. Let's inspire each other to be the best versions of ourselves and make this year a transformative one filled with growth, joy, and wellness. Together, we can achieve anything we set our minds to. Here's to a year of wellness, growth, and love!

Introduction

One Year Wellness Journey The Family Well-Being Edition is the smart guide for the health and happiness for the family. It is bad habit breaking, routine changing, self- discipline provoking information, draped in encouragement as well as enlightenment, resulting in continuous healing of the whole body. In this book, readers will embark on a comprehensive year-long journey that encompasses every aspect of wellness, including physical health, mental well-being, emotional balance, and spiritual growth. Each chapter focuses on a specific theme or area of wellness and provides valuable insights, challenges, and exercises to help readers make meaningful changes. The book offers a wide range of practical strategies to overcome obstacles, develop healthy habits, cultivate mindfulness, and enhance overall well-being. One Year Wellness Journey aims to empower readers to take charge of their well-being and achieve their wellness goals.

Over the course of a year, a family often encounters a wide range of experiences, challenges, and milestones. These may include celebrating holidays and special occasions together, navigating everyday routines and responsibilities, facing unexpected crises or emergencies, experiencing joys and sorrows, and adapting to changes such as moving to a new home, welcoming a new family member, or dealing with loss. Families may have to manage conflicts and disagreements, make important decisions together, support each other through difficult times, and celebrate achievements and successes. They may also encounter external factors such as economic fluctuations, health issues, work-related challenges, and social pressures. Overall, the family's collective experiences in a year shape their relationships, resilience, and growth, highlighting the importance of communication, understanding, and mutual support within the family unit.

Encounters: The Breakdown

1. Celebrations and Special Occasions: Birthdays, anniversaries, holidays, and other special events that bring the family together for joyous moments.

2. Everyday Routines and Responsibilities: Managing schedules, chores, school or work commitments, and other day-to-day tasks that keep the family functioning smoothly.

3. Unexpected Crises and Emergencies: Dealing with unforeseen challenges such as accidents, illnesses, natural disasters, or financial setbacks that require immediate attention and support.

4. Joys and Sorrows: Experiencing moments of happiness, laughter, and togetherness, as well as times of sadness, grief, and loss that impact the family's emotional well-being.

5. Changes and Transitions: Adjusting to significant life changes like moving to a new home, changing schools or jobs, welcoming a new family member, or coping with a separation or divorce.

6. Conflicts and Disagreements: Resolving disagreements, managing conflicts, and practicing effective communication to maintain harmony and understanding within the family.

7. Important Decisions: Making collective decisions about finances, education, healthcare, and other significant matters that affect the family's future and well-being.

8. Support Through Difficult Times: Providing emotional, practical, and moral support to each other during challenging periods like illness, loss, or personal struggles.

9. Achievements and Successes: Celebrating individual and collective accomplishments, milestones, and successes that bring pride and fulfillment to the family members.

10. External Factors and Pressures: Navigating external influences such as economic fluctuations, health issues, work-related challenges, social expectations, and cultural influences that impact the family dynamics and interactions.

Part 1: Physical Health

Chapter One: Jump-Starting a Healthy Lifestyle

Chapter One: Jump-Starting a Healthy Lifestyle

In the vast expanse of our daily lives, we often find ourselves forgetting to prioritize our well-being amidst the chaotic hustle and bustle. We rush from one task to another, neglecting the importance of nurturing our minds, bodies, and souls. However, within each of us lies the potential to embark on a transformative journey towards a healthier lifestyle, one that is brimming with vitality and joy.

To jump-start a healthy lifestyle, it begins with a shift in our mindset. We must first recognize and embrace the significance of self-care, understanding that our well-being is not a luxury but a necessity. This mental shift paves the way for us to embark on a holistic journey wherein we consciously choose to nourish our bodies and minds with nutritious foods, engaging activities, and positive thoughts.

Taking small, intentional steps is paramount in this journey towards wellness. It starts with fueling our bodies with wholesome, nutrient-rich foods that replenish our energy levels and support our physical and mental health. By incorporating a colorful variety of fruits, vegetables, lean proteins, and whole grains into our diet, we nourish our bodies from within, laying the foundation for vitality and strength.

Alongside a balanced and wholesome diet, physical activity forms an integral part of our pursuit of a healthier lifestyle. Regular exercise not only helps in maintaining a healthy weight but also releases endorphins, promoting an overall sense of happiness and well-being. Whether it's yoga sessions, brisk walks in nature, or engaging in a sport we enjoy, finding an activity that resonates with us encourages consistency and makes exercise a joyful habit rather than a dreaded chore.

Nurturing our mental health is equally important in our journey towards a healthier lifestyle. In a world where stress and anxiety often cloud our minds, it is essential to find moments of tranquility and peace. Through mindful practices such as meditation, journaling, or engaging in creative endeavors, we carve out space for self-reflection, allowing us to let go of negative thoughts and focus on the present moment, fostering inner peace and balance.

Moreover, an essential aspect of jump-starting a healthy lifestyle is fostering a supportive and encouraging environment. Surrounding ourselves with like-minded individuals who value wellness allows us to create a network of individuals who inspire and motivate each other. Sharing our goals, challenges, and victories with this community bolsters our commitment towards our own well-being and provides a safe space for growth.

As we embark on this journey towards a healthier lifestyle, it is crucial to remember that change takes time and patience. Small, consistent actions build the foundation for lasting habits and transformations. By prioritizing our health, embracing a positive mindset, nourishing our bodies, moving with purpose, and nurturing our mental well-being, we lay the groundwork for a life filled with vibrancy, energy, and fulfillment.

Seeing as were jump starting a healthy lifestyle, it involves going to the doctor to see where we are with our health. There are those that refuse to go to the doctor for anything. That we must address and understand before moving forward.

There are several reasons why people may feel hesitant or uncomfortable about going to the doctor. First and foremost, many individuals have a fear of receiving bad news or a serious diagnosis during a medical appointment. This fear of the unknown can lead to avoidance of doctor visits altogether. Additionally, some people may feel embarrassed or ashamed about their health concerns, especially if they are related to sensitive topics such as mental health, sexual health, or substance abuse. There may also be financial barriers that prevent individuals from seeking medical care, such as high healthcare costs or lack of insurance coverage. Furthermore, some individuals may have had negative experiences with healthcare providers in the past, leading to a lack of trust in the medical system. Should they go they don't ask questions.

When it comes to asking questions to doctors about their health, people may feel intimidated or overwhelmed by the medical jargon and complex information that doctors provide. This can result in individuals feeling unsure of how to ask meaningful questions or advocate for their own health needs. Additionally, some people may feel rushed or dismissed during medical appointments, leading them to believe that their questions are not important or valued by healthcare providers. Cultural factors can also play a role, as certain cultures may emphasize deference to authority figures like doctors, making it difficult for individuals to speak up and ask questions about their health. Overall, a combination of fear, embarrassment, lack of trust, communication barriers, and cultural factors can all contribute to why individuals may not feel comfortable asking doctors questions about their health.

Asking questions to your healthcare providers is an essential part of receiving quality healthcare and being an active participant in your own health management. It is important to seek clarification, gather information, and understand your health conditions, treatments, and options effectively. By asking questions, you can gain a better understanding of your health needs, make informed decisions about your care, and actively engage in discussions with your healthcare team. Feeling comfortable about asking questions creates a positive and collaborative relationship with your healthcare providers, leading to better communication and ultimately better health outcomes. Remember, your healthcare providers are there to help you, and they value your involvement and participation in your healthcare journey. So, don't hesitate to ask questions and advocate for yourself to ensure that you receive the best possible care tailored to your individual needs.

I understand that you may have reservations about visiting the doctor, but it is crucial to seek preventive healthcare and overall well-being. I want you to know the importance of early detection and proactive healthcare management in preventing serious health issues in the future. By getting the benefits of regular check-ups, screenings, and preventive care, you may be more motivated to prioritize your health and schedule routine medical appointments. I assure you that you can do it, and I support you. I pray that I can help alleviate your fears and anxieties associated with visiting the doctor. Once you make the first appointment, through open communication, empathy, and understanding from healthcare providers, as well as from family and friends, who can offer encouragement and accompany you to medical appointments if needed. Additionally, having a positive mindset towards healthcare can help in feeling more in control of health outcomes and more willing to seek medical advice and support when needed. Lastly, there are community resources that can address practical barriers such as financial concerns or lack of access to healthcare. Those resources can also help make seeking medical care more feasible and attainable for individuals who may be hesitant to visit the doctor. Let's be safe now rather than sorry later, go see about yourselves. This is the starting point for jump starting your healthy lifestyle.

Now that we know where we are physically, we can set some real fitness goals. Setting realistic fitness goals is crucial for several reasons. Firstly, realistic goals help to provide focus and motivation, giving individuals a clear target to work towards. This can make the fitness journey more manageable and less overwhelming. Additionally, setting achievable goals allows for a sense of accomplishment and progress, boosting confidence and morale along the way. It also helps individuals to track their progress effectively and make any adjustments to their fitness routine if necessary. Finally, realistic goals promote sustainability and long-term success in maintaining a healthy lifestyle, as they are more likely to be attainable and sustainable over time. Overall, setting realistic fitness goals is essential for fostering a positive mindset, staying motivated, and ultimately achieving optimal health and well-being.

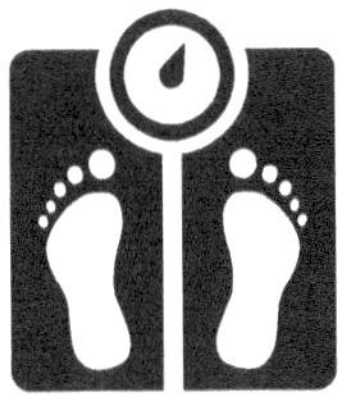

The Toll on The Physical

In the chaotic whirlwind of a modern lifestyle, it can be all too easy to succumb to unhealthy habits that take a toll on our physical health. An unhealthy lifestyle, encompassing poor dietary choices, sedentary behavior, inadequate sleep, and high levels of stress, contributes to a myriad of health issues. The effects ripple through our bodies, manifesting in weight gain, weakened immune systems, increased risk of chronic diseases such as heart disease and diabetes, reduced energy levels, and a decline in overall vitality. The lack of nutritious foods and overreliance on processed, sugary, and high-fat options leave our bodies starved for essential nutrients and susceptible to weight gain and inflammation. Coupled with a sedentary lifestyle that promotes prolonged sitting and lack of physical activity, our muscles weaken, our metabolism slows, and our risk of obesity and associated health conditions skyrockets. Insufficient sleep, often a consequence of a hectic and stress-filled life, further undermines our physical health, leaving us vulnerable to a compromised immune system, hormonal imbalances, and mood disturbances. The accumulating stress from work pressures, relationship strains, financial worries, and the constant demand of daily life also takes a harsh toll, releasing a flood of stress hormones that can damage our cardiovascular system, impair our mental health, and even contribute to premature aging. When we neglect the importance of a healthy lifestyle, our physical health inevitably suffers, compromising our ability to thrive and enjoy a life of well-being and vitality.

Living an unhealthy lifestyle can have detrimental effects on the body, mind, and spirit. Bad habits such as smoking and excessive drinking can lead to overall decreased physical health. Mentally, an unhealthy lifestyle can contribute to depression as the body struggles to cope with the negative effects. Spiritually, neglecting one's overall well-being can lead to a sense of disconnect from oneself and a lack of purpose or fulfillment. It is important to prioritize self-care and make positive choices for a balanced and healthy lifestyle to maintain overall well-being.

Undoing the toll of unhealthy habits on the body is a transformative journey that requires patience, determination, and self-love. It's never too late to start making positive changes towards a healthier lifestyle. By acknowledging the impact of your unhealthy habits and taking proactive steps to reverse their effects, you are choosing to prioritize your well-being and longevity. Whether it's quitting smoking, reducing alcohol consumption, getting regular exercise, or improving your diet, each small change you make is a step in the right direction. Remember, progress is not always linear, and setbacks may happen along the way. Be kind to yourself and celebrate the small victories, no matter how seemingly insignificant they may appear. Every healthy choice you make is a step towards healing and rejuvenating your body. With perseverance and a supportive mindset, you can undo the toll of unhealthy habits and embark on a path towards a healthier, happier, and more vibrant you. Your body has incredible resilience, and with your commitment to making positive changes, you have the power to reclaim your health and well-being.

Using a family health and fitness questionnaire is an effective way to determine the fitness goals of each family member and identify common goals as a family unit. The questionnaire can cover a range of topics such as current exercise habits, dietary preferences, overall health conditions, and individual fitness aspirations. By collecting this information, the family can assess their current health status, identify areas for improvement, and set specific, measurable goals that are tailored to their collective needs. This collaborative approach fosters accountability and motivation, allowing the family to work together towards achieving a healthier and more active lifestyle.

Family Health and Fitness Questionnaire:

1. How would you rate your current health and fitness level on a scale of 1 to 10 (1 being very poor, 10 being excellent)?

2. Do you currently engage in any physical activity or exercise on a regular basis? If yes, what type of activities do you participate in and how often?

3. How many hours of sleep do you typically get per night?

4. Do you have any existing medical conditions or health concerns that may impact your ability to exercise or maintain good health? If yes, please specify.

5. On a typical day, what does your diet consist of? (e.g., fruits/ vegetables, processed foods, sugary drinks)

6. How often does your family engage in physical activities or exercise together?

7. Are there any barriers or challenges that prevent you from maintaining a healthy lifestyle and regular exercise routine?

8. Do you have any specific health or fitness goals for yourself or your family members that you would like to achieve for the near future?

9. Have you or any family members previously consulted with a healthcare provider or fitness professional regarding your health and fitness goals?

10. What kind of support or resources would you find helpful in improving your family's health and fitness?

11. What are your fitness goals?

Going on a family wellness journey can be a truly transformative and empowering experience. By utilizing a family health and fitness questionnaire, you are provided the opportunity to gather valuable insights into each family member's health, fitness levels, and wellness goals. This collaborative effort not only helps create a clear roadmap for your fitness journey but also fosters a sense of unity and support within the family. Sharing your aspirations, challenges, and triumphs through this process can strengthen bonds and motivate each other to stay committed to your goals. Embrace this opportunity to prioritize your family's health and well-being together and watch how this shared commitment leads to a healthier, happier, and more connected family unit. Start your wellness journey today with the power of reflection, planning, and togetherness.

Having some trouble with the questions, here is an example of answers to a family health and fitness questionnaire:

1. How often do you engage in physical activity?

- Mom: I exercise 3 times a week, mostly running and yoga.

- Dad: I play basketball with friends twice a week and lift weights at home.

- Child 1: I have soccer practice 3 times a week.

- Child 2: I enjoy dancing and do it at least 4 times a week.

2. What are your current fitness goals?

- Mom: I want to improve my flexibility and core strength.

- Dad: I aim to increase my muscle mass and overall endurance.

- Child 1: I want to get faster and stronger for soccer games.

- Child 2: I just want to have fun and stay active.

3. Are there any health conditions or dietary restrictions we should be aware of?

- Mom: I have lactose intolerance and try to avoid dairy.

- Dad: I have high blood pressure, so I watch my salt intake.

- Child 1: I have a nut allergy and need to be mindful of what I eat.

- Child 2: I don't have any specific health issues but prefer vegetarian meals.

4. What motivates you to stay active and make healthy choices?

- Mom: I want to have more energy to keep up with my family and live a long, fulfilling life.

- Dad: I want to set a positive example for my kids and be able to participate in physical activities with them.

- Child 1: I love the feeling of accomplishment after a good workout and want to be the best player on my team.

- Child 2: I enjoy being active and it makes me feel happy and strong.

These answers provide a glimpse into each family member's habits, goals, and motivations, which can guide the family towards creating a personalized wellness plan that meets everyone's needs and aspirations. This is also a good time to open conversation about any new or preexisting health problems that should be taken into consideration. As well as answering any questions members have about family health history, we'll go into further detail in another chapter later.

After completing the family health and fitness questionnaire, the next step is to translate those insights into a realistic and achievable fitness plan tailored to the needs and goals of each family member. By analyzing the responses and identifying common themes and areas for improvement, the family can collaboratively design a plan that includes specific fitness activities, dietary adjustments, and lifestyle changes. This plan should be realistic, making an allowance for each family member's schedules, preferences, and abilities to ensure long-term adherence and success. Setting measurable goals, establishing a timeline, and incorporating strategies for accountability and support will help the family stay focused and motivated on their wellness journey. With a well-crafted fitness plan in place, the family is now equipped to take proactive steps towards improving their health and well-being as a unit. *At the end of the book, you will find a One Year Family Wellness Plan Worksheet to help your family keep track of your progress over the year journey.*

Ways for Setting Realistic Fitness Goals and Creating a Personalized Exercise Plan

1. Start with self-reflection: Begin by taking a moment to assess your current fitness level, lifestyle, and any specific health considerations you might have. Understand where you're starting from to set realistic and achievable goals.

2. Define your objectives: Clearly outline what you want to achieve through your fitness journey. Is it weight loss, increased muscle strength, cardiovascular endurance, or overall well-being? Having specific goals will provide direction and motivation to work towards.

3. Set SMART goals: Utilize the SMART goal-setting approach - Specific, Measurable, Achievable, Relevant, and Time-bound. Instead of simply aiming to "lose weight," set a specific target, such as "lose 10 pounds in three months by following a healthy diet and exercising three times a week." This approach makes your goals clear, measurable, and attainable.

4. Break it down: Divide your overarching goal into smaller, manageable milestones. This helps you track your progress and celebrate achievements along the way. For example, if your main goal is to run a marathon, break it down into smaller goals like running a certain distance each week or increasing your pace gradually.

5 Assess your time and resources: Consider the time and resources you have available to dedicate towards your fitness goals. Be realistic about how many days per week you can commit exercising and what equipment or facilities you have access to. Adapt your plan accordingly to fit your lifestyle.

6. Seek professional guidance: If you're unsure about creating a personalized exercise plan, consult with a fitness professional or personal trainer. They can help assess your needs, provide expert advice, and design a plan tailored to your goals and capabilities.

7. Choose activities you enjoy: Incorporate activities that you genuinely enjoy into your exercise plan. Whether it's dancing, swimming, hiking, or going to the gym, finding activities you look forward to will keep you motivated and engaged.

8. Mix it up: Avoid monotony by incorporating a variety of exercises and activities into your plan. This helps prevent boredom and keeps your body challenged, leading to better results over time. Consider combining cardio, strength training, and flexibility exercises for a well-rounded routine.

9. Listen to your body: Pay attention to how your body responds to exercise. Learn to distinguish between soreness from a good workout and pain that indicates an injury. Adjust your plan, accordingly, incorporating rest days and modifications to prevent overexertion and promote healthy recovery.

10. Monitor and adjust: Regularly track your progress and make all adjustments as needed. Keep a workout journal, use fitness apps, or consult with a professional to monitor your development. If you meet a milestone earlier than expected or realize a certain exercise is not working for you, adapt your plan accordingly.

Remember, setting realistic fitness goals requires patience, commitment, and a sustainable approach. Stay focused, celebrate your achievements, and embrace the journey towards a healthier, stronger, and more confident you.

There are many different exercises that are simple for the family and can be done by all your family members at any time. Let's take a glance.

Wall Pilates Exercises

Engaging in wall Pilates is a fantastic way to reap numerous physical and mental health benefits while also having a fun and effective workout experience. By incorporating the support of a wall into your Pilates routine, you can enhance your practice and target specific muscle groups with precision and control. The stability provided by the wall allows you to focus on proper alignment, deepen your stretches, and improve your overall posture. Additionally, wall Pilates can help build strength, flexibility, and balance, leading to improved core stability and muscle tone. This form of Pilates is suitable for practitioners of all levels, as the wall serves as a versatile prop that can be adjusted to accommodate different abilities and goals. Embracing wall Pilates also offers the opportunity to increase body awareness, mindfulness, and relaxation, making it a holistic practice that benefits both the body and mind. So, whether you are looking to enhance your physical fitness, correct imbalances, or simply add variety to your workout routine, trying wall Pilates can be a rewarding and rejuvenating experience that brings numerous benefits to your health and well-being. Get ready to challenge yourself, feel stronger, and enjoy the transformative effects of wall Pilates on your body and mind!

Wall Pilates exercises are a wonderful way to enhance your Pilates practice by utilizing the support and resistance of a wall to target specific muscle groups, improve alignment, and deepen stretches. Here are some popular wall Pilates exercises along with their benefits:

1. Wall Roll Down: Stand facing the wall with your feet hip-width apart and slowly roll down through the spine, utilizing the wall for support. This exercise helps to release tension in the spine, hamstrings, and calves while improving spinal mobility and posture.

2. Wall Squats: Stand with your back against the wall and lower into a squat position, keeping your knees aligned with your ankles. Wall squats are great for strengthening the quadriceps, glutes, and core muscles while promoting proper alignment and stability.

3. Wall Angels: Lie on the floor with your knees bent and feet against the wall, then slide your arms up and down the wall in a snow-angel motion. This exercise helps improve shoulder mobility, strengthen the upper back muscles, and open the chest.

4. Wall Plank: Begin in a plank position with your hands on the floor and feet against the wall, forming a straight line from head to heels. Wall planks challenge the core muscles, shoulders, and arms while also improving stability and balance.

5. Wall Bridge: Lie on your back with your feet on the wall and lift your hips towards the ceiling, engaging your glutes and core. Wall bridges are excellent for strengthening the glutes, hamstrings, and lower back muscles while improving hip mobility and stability.

Benefits of wall Pilates exercises include improved posture, increased strength and flexibility, enhanced core stability, better body awareness, reduced risk of injury, and a sense of relaxation and well-being. Incorporating these exercises into your Pilates routine can help you target specific muscle groups, deepen your stretches, and take your practice to the next level. Enjoy the benefits of wall Pilates and experience a stronger, more balanced body and mind!

Chair Pilates

Chair Pilates exercises are a fantastic way to incorporate the principles of Pilates into your daily routine, offering a convenient and effective way to improve strength, flexibility, and overall mobility. Here is a detailed list of chair Pilates exercises along with their benefits:

1. Chair Squats: Stand in front of a sturdy chair with feet hip-width apart and slowly lower into a squat position, engaging your core and glutes. Benefits include strengthening the quadriceps, hamstrings, and glutes, improving lower body strength, and enhancing balance and stability.

2. Seated Leg Extensions: Sit on the edge of a chair with your back straight and extend one leg in front of you, then lower it back down. This exercise targets the quadriceps and helps improve leg strength, flexibility, and range of motion.

3. Chair Plank: Place your hands on a chair seat and walk your feet back into a plank position, holding your body in a straight line. Chair planks engage the core, arms, and shoulders, helping to improve overall strength, stability, and balance.

4. Seated Spinal Twists: Sit tall in the chair and twist your torso to one side, then the other, gently stretching the spine and engaging the core muscles. Seated spinal twists help improve spinal mobility, release tension, and promote better posture.

5. Chair Leg Circles: Sit on the chair with one leg extended and circle the leg in a controlled motion, targeting the hip flexors and outer thighs. This exercise helps improve hip mobility, strengthen the thigh muscles, and enhance flexibility.

Benefits of chair Pilates exercises include improved posture, increased core strength, enhanced flexibility, better balance, and stability, reduced back pain, and enhanced body awareness. By incorporating these chair Pilates exercises into your daily routine, you can reap the numerous physical and mental benefits of Pilates in a convenient and accessible way. Enjoy the benefits of chair Pilates and experience a stronger, more flexible, and balanced body and mind!

Chair Pilates for the physically limited. No, you don't get left out of Pilates.

Chair Pilates exercises can be a great option for individuals with disabilities, providing a safe and accessible way to improve strength, flexibility, and overall well-being. Here is a detailed list of chair Pilates exercises that are specifically beneficial for individuals with disabilities, along with their corresponding benefits:

1. Seated Leg Extensions: Sitting tall in a chair, extending one leg at a time in front of you, flexing and pointing the foot. This exercise helps improve leg strength, flexibility, and range of motion, making it beneficial for individuals with mobility challenges.

2. Seated Torso Twists: Sit in a chair with your feet flat on the floor and gently rotate your torso from side to side, engaging your core muscles. Seated torso twists can help improve spinal mobility, relieve tension, and enhance overall body awareness.

3. Seated Leg Lifts: While seated, lift one leg at a time, engaging the quadriceps and core muscles. This exercise helps strengthen the lower body, improve balance, and enhance stability, making it beneficial for individuals with limited mobility in the lower extremities.

4. Seated Shoulder Rolls: Sit comfortably in a chair and roll your shoulders back and down in a circular motion. Seated shoulder rolls can help reduce shoulder tension, improve posture, and enhance upper body mobility, which can be particularly beneficial for individuals with mobility issues in the upper body.

5. Chair Plank Modifications: Place your hands on the seat of a chair and walk your feet back into a plank position, holding for a few seconds. Chair plank modifications can be adjusted to suit

individual abilities and can help strengthen the core, arms, and shoulders, promoting overall stability and balance.

Benefits of chair Pilates exercises for individuals with disabilities include improved muscle strength, enhanced flexibility, better posture, increased body awareness, reduced risk of injury, and boosted confidence and self-esteem. By incorporating these gentle and effective chair Pilates exercises into a regular routine, individuals with disabilities can experience the physical and mental benefits of Pilates in a safe and supportive environment. Enjoy the benefits of chair Pilates and promote a stronger, more flexible, and balanced body and mind, regardless of physical limitations.

Family Pilates is a wonderful way for families to bond, stay active together, and promote health and well-being as a unit. Participating in Pilates as a family can create a supportive and motivating environment in which everyone can work towards their fitness goals while enjoying quality time together. Family Pilates classes or sessions can be tailored to accommodate members of all ages and fitness levels, making it a fun and inclusive activity for everyone.

Parents can set a positive example for their children by prioritizing their own health and wellness, fostering a culture of fitness within the family. Children, in turn, can learn the importance of staying active, taking care of their bodies, and developing good posture and body awareness through Pilates exercises. Family Pilates sessions can also provide a platform for open communication, teamwork, and mutual encouragement, strengthening family relationships and promoting a sense of unity.

Pilates exercises can be adapted to suit the needs and abilities of each family member, making it a versatile and accessible activity for all. From gentle stretches and breathing exercises to more challenging core-strengthening movements, there is a wide range of Pilates exercises that can be enjoyed by the whole family. By engaging in these exercises together, family members can support each other, celebrate progress, and share in the satisfaction of achieving fitness goals as a team.

In addition to the physical benefits of improved strength, flexibility, and posture, family Pilates can also bring about mental and emotional benefits such as reduced stress, increased mindfulness, and a sense of accomplishment. Creating a routine of regular family Pilates sessions can instill healthy habits, promote positive lifestyle choices, and enhance overall well-being for every family member.

Ultimately, family Pilates is a holistic and enjoyable way for families to connect, prioritize their health, and embark on a journey towards improved physical and mental wellness together. By incorporating Pilates into your family's routine, you can foster a supportive and health-conscious environment that promotes unity, strength, and vitality for all. So, give it a go and see how things can change for the family.

Another way for families to repair the damage from the physical toll is to have family yoga sessions. You all can take classes outside or inside the home.

Family yoga is a beautiful and rewarding practice that promotes connection, mindfulness, and physical wellness among family members of all ages. Bringing together the ancient practice of yoga and the bond of family, family yoga sessions create a nurturing and supportive environment where parents and children can practice together, share experiences, and grow together on and off the mat.

Family yoga classes typically incorporate a mix of traditional yoga poses, breathing exercises, relaxation techniques, and playful activities that cater to the needs and interests of all family members. From gentle stretches to dynamic movements, family yoga sessions offer a holistic approach to health and well-being that benefits the body, mind, and spirit.

Participating in family yoga can strengthen the family bond, foster communication, and build trust and cooperation among family members. Parents can lead by example, demonstrating the importance of self-care, mindfulness, and physical activity to their children. Children, in turn, can learn valuable skills such as focus, balance, and emotional regulation through the practice of yoga.

Family yoga is a versatile practice that can be adapted to suit the abilities and preferences of each family member, making it inclusive and accessible to everyone. Whether practicing calming breathing exercises, engaging in partner poses, or enjoying relaxing meditation, family yoga sessions provide a space for creativity, self-expression, and shared experiences that nourish the body, mind, and soul.

In addition to the physical benefits of increased strength, flexibility, and balance, family yoga also offers a range of mental and emotional benefits. Practicing mindfulness and relaxation techniques together can reduce stress, improve concentration, and promote a sense of calm and well-being among family members.

By incorporating family yoga into your routine, you can cultivate a sense of togetherness, health, and harmony within your family. Through the practice of yoga, families can create lasting memories, strengthen relationships, and embark on a journey of self-discovery and growth together. Family yoga is a beautiful opportunity to connect, center, and thrive as a family unit, creating a foundation of health and happiness that extends beyond the mat.

How to have in home family Yoga

To engage in family yoga and incorporate this wonderful practice into your family routine, consider the following steps to create a fun and meaningful experience for all family members:

1. Establish a Dedicated Space: Designate a quiet and clutter-free area in your home where you can practice family yoga together. Ensure there is enough space for everyone to move freely and comfortably. Consider adding calming elements such as candles, cushions, or soothing music to create a peaceful atmosphere.

2. Schedule Regular Sessions: Set aside dedicated time in your family's schedule for yoga practice. Whether it's a few times a week or once a month, consistency is key to incorporating family yoga into your routine. Choose a time that works for everyone and commit to making it a priority.

3. Plan Family-Friendly Sequences: Research family-friendly yoga poses and sequences that cater to the abilities and interests of all family members. Incorporate a mix of standing, seated, and lying-down poses, as well as breathing exercises and relaxation techniques. Encourage creativity and self-expression during practice.

4. Make it Interactive and Fun: Include playful and engaging activities in your family yoga sessions to keep everyone interested and involved. Try partner poses, animal-inspired poses, or storytelling through movement to make the practice enjoyable for children and adults alike. Encourage laughter and exploration as you move through the sequence together.

5. Focus on Mindfulness and Connection: Encourage mindfulness and presence during the practice by guiding family members to focus on their breath, sensations in their body, and the present moment. Encourage open communication, empathy, and mutual support among family members as you practice together.

6. Embrace Flexibility and Adaptation: Be open to adapting the practice based on the needs and abilities of each family member. Offer modifications for poses, provide options for challenges, and

foster a spirit of acceptance and non-judgment within your family yoga practice.

7. Reflect and Celebrate: After each family yoga session, take a moment to reflect on your experience together. Celebrate your accomplishments, express gratitude for the opportunity to practice as a family and discuss any insights or feelings that arose during the practice. Encourage open dialogue and connection among family members.

By following these steps and incorporating family yoga into your routine, you can create a nurturing, engaging, and joyful practice that promotes health, connection, and well-being within your family. Family yoga is a beautiful opportunity to bond, grow, and thrive together, fostering a sense of unity, strength, and harmony among family members.

Family Yoga Poses

Here is a list of family yoga poses that can be enjoyed together with children and adults. These poses are fun, interactive, and suitable for practitioners of all ages and abilities:

1. Partner Tree Pose

- Stand side by side with your partner, holding hands for balance.

- Lift one foot and place the sole against the inner thigh of the standing leg.

- Lift the arms overhead and find a focal point to help with balance.

- Hold the pose for several breaths and then switch sides.

2. Duo Downward Dog

- Start in a downward facing dog pose.

- Have one family member walk their feet towards the hands of the other family member.

- The person in front will hold the other person's ankles for support.

- Both partners maintain the downward dog position, stretching the back and legs.

3. Parent-Child Boat Pose

- Sit facing each other with your knees bent and feet flat on the floor.

- Hold hands and lean back, engaging the core muscles.

- Lift your feet off the ground, finding balance in boat pose.

- Hold the pose while maintaining eye contact and smiling at each other.

4. Family Windmill Twist

- Sit cross-legged in a circle with your family members, holding hands.

- Inhale to lengthen the spine, then exhale and twist to one side, following the movement of your family members.

- Inhale back to center, then exhale and twist to the other side.

- Repeat the twisting motion in sync with your family members, creating a flowing movement.

5. Group Butterfly Pose

- Sit in a circle with the soles of your feet touching, forming a diamond shape with your legs.

- Hold hands with your family members and gently flap your "butterfly wings" by moving your knees up and down.

- Encourage a gentle bounce as you connect with your family members in this heart-opening pose.

6. Partner Forward Fold

- Sit facing your partner with your feet touching.

- Reach for each other's hands and slowly fold forward, keeping the spine long.

- Allow the head to hang heavy and feel a gentle stretch in the hamstrings and back.

- Breathe deeply and relax into the pose together.

These family yoga poses promote connection, communication, and shared experiences while nurturing the body and mind. Enjoy practicing these poses with your loved ones and have fun exploring the benefits of family yoga together.

Walking

Walking is a fantastic form of exercise that offers numerous benefits for both physical and mental health. It is a simple yet effective way to improve overall health and well-being for individuals of all ages. The following is a detailed explanation of the benefits of walking for better health for you and your family:

Benefits of Walking for Better Health:

1. Cardiovascular Health: Walking helps to improve cardiovascular health by increasing heart rate and strengthening the heart muscle. It also helps to lower blood pressure and reduce the risk of heart disease and stroke.

2. Weight Management: Regular walking can help with weight management by burning calories and boosting metabolism. It can also help to tone muscles and improve overall body composition.

3. Improved Mood: Walking has been shown to boost mood and reduce symptoms of anxiety and depression. It helps to release endorphins, the body's natural "feel-good" chemicals, which can improve mental well-being.

4. Boosted Immune System: Regular walking can strengthen the immune system, making you less susceptible to illnesses and infections.

5. Joint Health: Walking is a low-impact exercise that can help improve joint health and reduce the risk of arthritis and other joint-related conditions.

6. Increased Energy Levels: Walking can increase energy levels and combat feelings of fatigue. It can also improve sleep quality, leading to better overall energy and productivity.

7. Social Benefits: Walking can be a social activity that allows you and your family to spend quality time together while improving their health. It can foster connections and strengthen relationships.

Benefits for You and Your Family:

1. Family Bonding: Walking as a family provides an opportunity to bond, communicate, and enjoy quality time together. It can strengthen relationships and create lasting memories.

2. Improved Health: Walking can improve the overall health and well-being of each family member, reducing the risk of various health conditions and promoting longevity.

3. Stress Relief: Walking can be a great way for the whole family to de-stress and unwind after a long day. It can provide a break from daily routines and offer mental refreshment.

4. Role Modeling: By engaging in regular walking as a family, you can serve as a positive role model for your children and encourage them to adopt healthy habits from a young age.

5. Outdoor Time: Walking outdoors allows the family to enjoy fresh air, sunlight, and nature, which can have additional benefits for mental health and overall well-being.

The number of miles you should aim to walk per day can vary depending on your fitness level, health goals, and lifestyle. Generally, experts recommend getting at least 150 minutes of moderate-intensity exercise per week, such as walking, which amounts to about 7-10,000 steps per day or roughly 3-5 miles for most adults. Here is a detailed explanation of why walking a certain number of miles per day makes a difference in your overall health and fitness:

Why Walking Miles Per Day Makes a Difference:

1. Cardiovascular Fitness: Walking several miles per day can help improve cardiovascular fitness by strengthening the heart muscle, increasing circulation, and improving overall heart health. This can result in a reduced risk of heart disease and stroke.

2. Weight Management: Walking a certain number of miles per day can aid in weight management by burning calories and increasing metabolism. Consistently meeting a daily walking goal can help with weight loss or maintenance and improve body composition.

3. Improved Endurance: Regular walking can enhance endurance and stamina, allowing you to engage in physical activities for longer periods without feeling fatigued. This can lead to better overall fitness levels.

4. Muscle Strength: Walking several miles per day can help tone and strengthen muscles, particularly in the legs, hips, and core. This can improve balance, stability, and overall strength.

5. Bone Health: Weight-bearing activities like walking are beneficial for bone health and can help prevent osteoporosis by increasing bone density and strength.

6. Mental Health: Walking can have positive effects on mental health by reducing stress and anxiety, improving mood, and boosting self-esteem. Achieving a daily walking goal can provide a sense of accomplishment and well-being.

7. Overall, Health Benefits: Walking a certain number of miles per day can have a wide range of health benefits, including improved immune function, better sleep quality, reduced risk of chronic diseases like diabetes and hypertension, and enhanced overall well-being.

8. Consistency and Habit Formation: Setting a daily walking goal can help establish a consistent exercise routine and create healthy habits. Regular physical activity is key to maintaining good health and fitness.

In summary, walking is a simple yet powerful form of exercise that offers a wide range of benefits for both individuals and families. By combining walks into your routine, you can improve your health, bond with your loved ones, and create a positive and healthy lifestyle for your family. Walking a certain number of miles per day can have a significant impact on your overall health and fitness. Setting and achieving a daily walking goal can improve cardiovascular fitness, aid in weight management, strengthen muscles, enhance endurance, and provide numerous mental health benefits. By incorporating regular walks into your daily routine, you can enjoy a healthier and more active lifestyle.

Chapter Two: Nurturing Your Body

49

Chapter Two: Nurturing Your Body

In the grand blueprint of life, our bodies are the vessels that carry us through every adventure, challenge, and triumph. Nurturing our bodies is an essential aspect of cultivating a healthier and more fulfilling existence. In this chapter, we explore the various dimensions of nurturing our physical selves - from the foods we consume to the movement we engage in, and even the rest and care we provide.

At the core of nurturing our bodies is the foundation of nutrition. By fueling our bodies with nutrient-dense and wholesome foods, we provide the building blocks for optimal health and vitality. Embracing a balanced and varied diet, rich in fruits, vegetables, whole grains, lean proteins, and healthy fats, supports our bodily functions, boosts our immune system, promotes weight management, and reduces the risk of chronic diseases. We delve into the importance of mindful eating, understanding portion control, and making informed choices to nourish our bodies from within.

Moving beyond the realm of nutrition, we explore the significance of movement and physical activity in nurturing our bodies. From gentle stretching to invigorating workouts, engaging in regular exercise not only strengthens our muscles and improves our physical fitness, but it also releases endorphins, uplifting our mood and enhancing our overall well-being. We discuss the importance of finding activities that inspire and challenge us, whether it be hiking, dancing, swimming, or any other form of movement that brings us joy. We also explore the benefits of incorporating resistance training, cardiovascular exercise, and flexibility workouts into our routine, creating a well-rounded approach to nurturing our bodies.

Furthermore, we delve into the critical component of rest and self-care. Prioritizing sleep and relaxation are essential in nurturing our bodies. Quality sleep allows our bodies to repair, rejuvenate, and replenish, enhancing our cognitive function, emotional well-being, and physical recovery. We discuss practical tips on creating a sleep-friendly environment and establishing healthy sleep habits. Additionally, we explore the importance of taking time for self-care activities, including practices such as massage, meditation, or simply indulging in activities that bring us joy and relaxation. Taking care of our bodies involves finding balance, allowing ourselves to rest and recharge amidst the demands of daily life.

By nurturing our physical selves through mindful nutrition, regular physical activity, and prioritizing rest and self-care, we pave the way for a life filled with vitality, strength, and overall well-being. In this chapter, we delve into the nuances of each dimension, providing practical tips and guidance to help us cultivate a nurturing relationship with our bodies, fostering a foundation for a healthier and happier life.

A healthful fluid intake

Proper hydration is essential for maintaining overall health and well-being across all age groups. Here is a detailed list of healthy fluid intake recommendations, alongside some refreshing drink ideas suitable for individuals of all ages:

Water:

1. Aim to drink at least 8-10 cups of water per day.

2. Keep a reusable water bottle handy to sip on throughout the day.

3. Flavor water with slices of citrus fruits, cucumber, or mint for added taste.

Herbal Teas:

1. Herbal teas are caffeine-free and can help hydrate the body.

2. Enjoy a warm cup of chamomile tea before bedtime for relaxation.

3. Herbal iced teas with berries or citrus slices are a refreshing summer drink option.

Smoothies:

1. Blend fruits like bananas, berries, and spinach with almond milk or coconut water for a hydrating and nutrient-packed drink.

2. Add a scoop of protein powder or Greek yogurt for added protein content.

3. Try a tropical smoothie with pineapple, mango, and coconut water for a taste of the tropics.

Coconut Water:

1. Coconut water is a natural electrolyte-rich beverage that can help replenish hydration levels.

2. Enjoy coconut water as a post-workout drink to rehydrate and replenish essential minerals.

3. Blend coconut water with fresh fruit for a hydrating and delicious smoothie option.

Green Juices:

1. Green juices made with leafy greens like spinach, kale, and cucumber are a great way to boost hydration levels and nutrient intake.

2. Add a splash of lemon or ginger for added flavor and cleansing benefits.

3. Enjoy green juice as a mid-morning or mid-afternoon pick-me-up.

Incorporating a variety of hydrating beverages into your daily routine and staying mindful of your fluid intake, you can support optimal health and hydration levels for individuals of all ages. Stay refreshed and nourished with these healthy drink ideas!

Now that we know some of the drink ideas, what are the benefits of a healthy fluid intake and how often should we hydrate? We don't want to overdo it. Everything in moderation, right? Yes.

Fluid intake: Summary and Benefits

Summary:

Proper fluid intake is essential for maintaining overall health and well-being for individuals of all ages. Water is the most crucial nutrient for the human body, as it is involved in almost every bodily function. Encouraging adequate fluid intake within a family can lead to numerous health benefits throughout the year. From improved hydration to better physical performance and cognitive function, staying properly hydrated can positively impact every aspect of one's life.

Benefits of fluid intake for a family in a year:

1. Hydration: Adequate fluid intake helps maintain proper hydration levels, which is essential for optimal bodily functions, such as temperature regulation and nutrient transport.

2. Energy levels: Staying hydrated can boost energy levels and reduce fatigue, helping family members stay active and engaged in daily activities.

3. Digestive health: Proper hydration supports digestion and helps prevent constipation, promoting overall gastrointestinal health for the entire family.

4. Skin health: Drinking enough fluids can improve skin hydration and elasticity, reducing the risk of dryness and skin issues for family members.

5. Weight management: Adequate fluid intake can aid in weight management by promoting satiety and reducing the likelihood of consuming excess calories from sugary beverages.

6. Kidney function: Proper hydration supports kidney function by helping to flush out waste products and prevent kidney stones, promoting optimal kidney health in family members.

7. Cognitive function: Staying hydrated is crucial for maintaining cognitive function, concentration, and overall brain health, benefiting family members of all ages.

8. Immune system support: Adequate fluid intake can help strengthen the immune system, potentially reducing the risk of infections and promoting overall health and well-being for the family.

9. Physical performance: Proper hydration can improve physical performance and endurance, allowing family members to engage in sports, exercise, and other physical activities with greater ease.

10. Mood and mental health: Hydration plays a role in maintaining mood stability and mental well-being, contributing to a more positive and productive family environment throughout the year.

Overall, encouraging and practicing adequate fluid intake as a family also facilitates the detoxification processes, regulates body temperature, supports healthy skin, hair, and nails which all lead to a wide range of health benefits and contribute to improved quality of life for everyone involved.

How many liters of water should I drink per day, based on general guidelines?

The general guideline for daily water intake is about 3.7 liters (or approximately 13 cups) for men and about 2.7 liters (or approximately 9 cups) for women. However, individual water needs can vary depending on factors such as age, activity level, and climate. It's always a good idea to listen to your body and drink water when you feel thirsty. Additionally, you may need to adjust your water intake based on your specific circumstances.

Staying adequately hydrated by consuming an optimal number of fluids offers numerous benefits for the entire family throughout the year. Hydration supports overall health and well-being by regulating body temperature, aiding digestion, and promoting proper organ function. It can also help prevent dehydration, which can lead to fatigue, headaches, and poor concentration. Proper fluid intake supports cognitive function and improves focus, helping both children and adults perform better in school, work, and daily activities. Hydration is essential for physical performance and exercise recovery, enhancing endurance and reducing the risk of muscle cramps and injuries. Additionally, maintaining optimal hydration levels supports healthy skin, hair, and nails, contributing to a vibrant appearance and boosting confidence. Regular fluid intake aids in the detoxification processes of the body, flushing out toxins and waste products. Moreover, staying hydrated can help prevent urinary tract infections and kidney stones, promote weight management by curbing hunger, and support immune function by keeping mucous membranes moist. Overall, prioritizing fluid intake as a family lead to improved health, energy levels, focus, and well-being throughout the year.

Drink more water!

The Basis of Healthy Eating for all.

A healthy diet is essential for overall well-being and longevity regardless of age. The foundation of a healthy diet includes a balanced intake of macronutrients such as carbohydrates, proteins, and fats, as well as a variety of micronutrients like vitamins and minerals. For individuals of all ages, it is crucial to focus on consuming whole, nutrient-dense foods such as fruits, vegetables, whole grains, lean proteins, and healthy fats. Meal ideas that incorporate these elements could include a colorful salad with mixed greens, cherry tomatoes, grilled chicken, avocado, and a balsamic vinaigrette dressing for lunch. For dinner, a well-rounded meal could consist of baked salmon with quinoa and roasted vegetables like carrots, broccoli, and sweet potatoes. Snacks like Greek yogurt with berries or a handful of nuts can provide additional nutrients and satisfy hunger between meals. Remember, consistency and moderation are key components of maintaining a healthy diet regardless of age.

Ready set let's go! Here is a list of healthy meal ideas suitable for individuals of all ages, along with some delicious dessert options:

Breakfast:

1. Greek yogurt parfait with layers of Greek yogurt, mixed berries, and granola

2. Whole grain toast with avocado slices and poached eggs

3. Overnight oats with almond butter, banana slices, and a sprinkle of cinnamon

Lunch:

1. Quinoa salad with chickpeas, roasted vegetables, feta cheese, and a lemon vinaigrette

2. Turkey and vegetable wrap with whole grain tortilla, hummus, and fresh greens

3. Lentil soup with a side of whole grain crackers and a mixed green salad

Dinner:

1. Baked teriyaki chicken with brown rice and steamed broccoli

2. Grilled shrimp skewers with quinoa tabbouleh and roasted asparagus

3. Vegetarian stir-fry with tofu, bell peppers, snap peas, and a soy-ginger sauce served over brown rice

Dessert:

1. Fresh fruit salad with a drizzle of honey and a sprinkle of nuts

2. Greek yogurt popsicles made with blended berries and a touch of honey

3. Dark chocolate-dipped strawberries or banana slices

4. Chia seed pudding with coconut milk and sliced almonds

Remember, incorporating a variety of whole foods and staying mindful of portion sizes can help maintain a balanced and healthy diet for individuals of all ages. Enjoy these meal ideas and treat yourself to a nutritious dessert as a satisfying end to your day!

Calorie Intake

How many calories should I eat per day, based on general guidelines?

The recommended daily caloric intake can vary based on factors such as age, gender, weight, height, and activity level. However, a general guideline for adults is around 2,000 to 2,500 calories per day for women and 2,500 to 3,000 calories per day for men to maintain weight. It's important to keep in mind that these are rough estimates and individual calorie needs may vary. If you are looking to lose weight, you may need to consume fewer calories, while if you are looking to gain weight, you may need to consume more. It's best to consult with a healthcare provider or a registered dietitian for personalized recommendations based on your specific needs and goals.

Here is an example of a day of meals totaling around 2,000 calories for a woman:

- Breakfast:

- 2 scrambled eggs (140 calories)

- 1 slice of whole grain toast (80 calories)

- 1 medium banana (105 calories)

- Mid-Morning Snack:

- 1 small Greek yogurt (100g) (100 calories)

- Lunch:

- Grilled chicken breast (150g) (220 calories)

- Mixed green salad with veggies and balsamic vinaigrette (150 calories)

- Afternoon Snack:

- 1 small apple (95 calories)

- 1 tablespoon of almond butter (90 calories)

- Dinner:

- Baked salmon (150g) (300 calories)

- Quinoa (1/2 cup) (111 calories)

- Steamed broccoli (80g) (35 calories)

- Evening Snack:

- Air-popped popcorn (1 cup) (30 calories)

This example provides a balanced mix of protein, healthy fats, whole grains, and fruits/vegetables while staying within the calorie range. Remember to adjust portion sizes and food choices based on your individual calorie needs and preferences. It's always a good idea to listen to your body's hunger and fullness cues and adjust accordingly.

Nutrition and a Balanced Diet

Nutrition is the process by which our body takes in and utilizes nutrients from the food we eat to maintain health and function properly. A balanced diet is essential for providing our bodies with the necessary nutrients they need to thrive. A balanced diet consists of a variety of foods from different food groups, including fruits, vegetables, whole grains, lean proteins, and healthy fats. Each of these food groups provides different vitamins, minerals, and essential macronutrients like carbohydrates, proteins, and fats that are vital for overall health. It is important to consume a variety of foods to ensure that our bodies receive a broad range of nutrients. A balanced diet can help prevent chronic diseases, maintain a healthy weight, support immunity, and promote overall well-being. Eating a balanced diet can have a significant impact on our energy levels, mood, and long-term health outcomes.

An acronym for diet. "D.I.N.E" which stands for Daily Intake and Nutritional Excellence.

Power Foods

1. Blueberries: Packed with antioxidants and phytochemicals, blueberries are known to support brain health, improve memory, and reduce the risk of chronic diseases like heart disease and cancer.

2. Spinach: Rich in vitamins A, C, and K, as well as iron and folate, spinach is a nutrient-dense leafy green that can promote bone health, improve digestion, and support a healthy immune system.

3. Salmon: An excellent source of omega-3 fatty acids, salmon is known for its heart-healthy benefits, as well as its ability to reduce inflammation, support brain function, and promote healthy skin and hair.

4. Quinoa: A complete protein source, quinoa is high in fiber, iron, and magnesium. It can help regulate blood sugar levels, support digestion, and provide sustained energy throughout the day.

5. Almonds: Packed with healthy fats, fiber, and protein, almonds are a nutrient-dense nut that can help lower cholesterol, reduce the risk of heart disease, and support brain function.

6. Greek Yogurt: High in protein and probiotics, Greek yogurt is beneficial for gut health, digestion, and immune function. It also provides essential nutrients like calcium and vitamin D for bone health.

These power foods are nutrient-dense and offer a wide range of health benefits, including improving overall health, reducing the risk of chronic diseases, and supporting vital bodily functions. Incorporating these foods into a balanced diet can help optimize health and well-being.

Energy Foods

1. Bananas: Packed with natural sugars, fiber, and essential nutrients like potassium and vitamin B6, bananas are a great source of quick energy. They can help replenish energy levels, support muscle function, and aid in digestion.

2. Oats: High in complex carbohydrates and fiber, oats provide a sustained release of energy throughout the day. They can help stabilize blood sugar levels, support heart health, and promote feelings of fullness and satiety.

3. Sweet Potatoes: Rich in carbohydrates, fiber, and vitamins A and C, sweet potatoes are a nutrient-dense energy food. They provide a steady source of energy, support immune function, and help regulate blood sugar levels.

4. Chia Seeds: Packed with omega-3 fatty acids, fiber, and protein, chia seeds can help boost energy levels, support digestion, and promote feelings of fullness. They also aid in hydration and can improve athletic performance.

5. Lentils: A good source of complex carbohydrates, protein, and fiber, lentils provide sustained energy and support muscle growth and repair. They are also rich in iron, which is essential for energy production and reducing fatigue.

6. Oranges: High in vitamin C and natural sugars, oranges are a refreshing energy booster. They can help improve immune function, support hydration, and provide a source of natural energy.

These energy foods are rich in carbohydrates, fiber, and essential nutrients that can provide a quick boost of energy as well as sustained energy throughout the day. Incorporating these foods into your diet can help fuel your body, improve performance, and support overall health and well-being.

Healing Foods

1. Bone Broth: Rich in collagen, amino acids, and minerals, bone broth is known for its healing properties. It can support gut health, reduce inflammation, boost immunity, and promote healthy skin, hair, and nails.

2. Ginger: A powerful anti-inflammatory and antioxidant, ginger has been used for centuries for its medicinal properties. It can help alleviate digestive issues, reduce pain and inflammation, support immune function, and improve circulation.

3. Turmeric: Contains the active compound curcumin, turmeric is a potent anti-inflammatory and antioxidant spice. It can help reduce inflammation, support joint health, boost immunity, aid in digestion, and promote overall well-being.

4. Honey: Known for its antimicrobial and healing properties, honey is a natural sweetener with numerous health benefits. It can soothe sore throats, alleviate coughs, promote wound healing, and support digestive health.

5. Fermented Foods: Foods like sauerkraut, kimchi, and kombucha are rich in probiotics that support gut health and digestion. Fermented foods can help balance the gut microbiome, boost immunity, and reduce inflammation.

6. Garlic: Contains sulfur compounds with antimicrobial and immune-boosting properties, garlic is a powerful healing food. It can help combat infections, lower cholesterol, reduce blood pressure, and support cardiovascular health.

These healing foods are rich in antioxidants, anti-inflammatory compounds, vitamins, and minerals that can support the body's natural healing processes, reduce inflammation, boost immunity, and promote overall health and well-being. Incorporating these foods into your diet can help nourish your body and support optimal health.

The power of nutrition and a balanced diet cannot be overstated when it comes to promoting overall health and well-being. Eating a variety of nutrient-dense foods from different food groups provides our bodies with the essential vitamins, minerals, and macronutrients needed to function optimally. A balanced diet can support a strong immune system, healthy weight maintenance, improved energy levels, and reduced risk of chronic diseases. Good nutrition can also have a profound impact on mental health, mood, and cognitive function. By fueling our bodies with the right combination of foods, we can enhance our quality of life and longevity. Making informed food choices and prioritizing a balanced diet is a powerful tool for achieving and maintaining optimal health in the long run.

Improving your nutrition and starting a balanced diet is a wonderful and empowering step towards a healthier and happier life. By making thoughtful choices about the foods you eat, you are giving your body the essential nutrients it needs to thrive. Remember, small changes can make a big difference. Start by incorporating more fruits, vegetables, whole grains, and lean proteins into your meals. Experiment with different recipes and cooking methods to make healthy eating exciting and enjoyable. Don't forget to stay hydrated and limit your consumption of processed foods and sugary drinks. Your body will thank you for nourishing it with wholesome, nutrient-rich foods. With dedication and a positive mindset, you can achieve your goal of improving your nutrition and embracing a balanced diet. Your health is worth the effort, so take the first step today towards a happier and healthier you!

Strategies for Improving Nutrition and Creating a Balanced Diet

1. Assess your current eating habits: Start by evaluating your current eating patterns. Take note of any unhealthy habits or areas where you could make improvements. This self-awareness will provide a foundation for creating a balanced diet.

2. Focus on whole foods: Emphasize whole, unprocessed foods in your diet. These include fruits, vegetables, whole grains, lean proteins, and healthy fats. Whole foods provide a wide range of essential nutrients, fiber, and antioxidants.

3. Portion control: Be mindful of portion sizes and aim for moderation. Even healthy foods can contribute to weight gain if consumed in excessive amounts. Use measuring tools or your hand as a guide to portion sizes and remember that listening to your body's hunger and fullness cues is crucial.

4. Incorporate variety: Aim for a colorful and diverse range of fruits and vegetables. Different colors provide different nutrients, so aim to include a variety of options in your meals. Experiment with new recipes and flavors to keep your meals exciting and nutritious.

5. Plan and prepare meals ahead of time: Set aside time each week to plan and prepare your meals. This reduces the reliance on processed or convenience foods and ensures you have nutritious options readily available. Prepare larger batches of healthy meals that can be stored and eaten throughout the week.

6. Limit added sugars and processed foods: Reduce your intake of added sugars, sugary beverages, and processed foods. These items often lack essential nutrients and can contribute to health issues like weight gain, diabetes, and heart disease.

7. Read food labels: Learn to read and understand food labels. Be aware of the ingredients, serving sizes, and nutritional information. This will help you make informed decisions and choose healthier options.

8. Hydration is key: Drink plenty of water throughout the day to stay properly hydrated. Water is essential for digestion, nutrient absorption, and overall well-being. Aim to drink at least eight glasses of water per day and adjust accordingly based on your activity level and climate.

9. Practice mindful eating: Slow down and savor your meals by practicing mindful eating. Pay attention to your body's hunger and fullness cues. This allows you to enjoy your food, appreciate the flavors, and prevent overeating.

10. Seek professional advice: Consider consulting with a registered dietitian or nutritionist who can provide personalized guidance based on your specific needs and goals. They can help you create

a balanced meal plan, address nutritional deficiencies, and offer ongoing support.

Bear in mind, improving nutrition and creating a balanced diet is a gradual process. Aim for progress, not perfection. Small, sustainable changes over time will lead to significant improvements in your overall health and well-being.

Nurturing the body goes beyond simply what we consume; it also involves how we care for our physical well-being. While maintaining a balanced and nutritious diet is crucial for good health, other factors play a significant role in nurturing the body. Nurturing the body encompasses more than just the food and drinks we consume; it also involves self-care practices that prioritize our physical and emotional well-being. Self-care is an essential aspect of nurturing the body, as it involves taking the time to engage in activities that promote relaxation, reduce stress, and enhance overall health. This can include activities such as exercise, meditation, spending time in nature, practicing mindfulness, getting regular massages, or engaging in hobbies that bring joy and fulfillment. Self-care helps to recharge our physical and emotional batteries, improving our resilience to stress and boosting our overall well-being. By incorporating self-care practices into our daily routine, we can better nurture our bodies and cultivate a positive relationship with ourselves, leading to greater levels of health and happiness in the long run.

Self-care

Caring for self is a great thing so embrace it.

- Exploring ways to prioritize self-care and promoting a positive body image

In a world that often places unrealistic expectations on appearance and fosters a culture of self-criticism, it becomes crucial to prioritize self-care and cultivate a positive body image. This chapter delves into the exploration of various strategies and practices that help us embrace self-compassion, nurture our minds and bodies, and foster a healthy relationship with ourselves.

One of the fundamental pillars of prioritizing self-care and promoting a positive body image is practicing self-acceptance and self-love. It begins with acknowledging and appreciating our unique qualities, focusing on our strengths rather than fixating on perceived flaws. We delve into the power of positive affirmations, mindfulness techniques, and gratitude practices, as they help shift our mindset and cultivate self-compassion.

Moreover, identifying and engaging in activities that bring us joy and fulfillment contributes to our overall well-being and self-care. Whether it's painting, dancing, practicing yoga, or spending time in nature, dedicating regular moments to engage in activities that nourish our souls allows us to reconnect with ourselves and promote a positive sense of self.

Another essential aspect is fostering a healthy body image. We explore the detrimental impact of societal pressures and unrealistic beauty standards and discuss strategies to challenge and overcome them. Developing a healthy body image starts with shifting our focus from external appearances to the incredible things our bodies are capable of. By emphasizing functionality, strength, and well-being, rather than conforming to stereotypical ideals, we can develop a greater appreciation for our bodies and prioritize self-care from a place of love and respect.

Furthermore, we address the importance of surrounding ourselves with a supportive community that uplifts and celebrates diversity. Building connections with individuals who value and encourage self-care and positive body image allows for a safe space to share experiences, challenges, and triumphs. We discuss the value of seeking professional help, such as therapy or counseling, if needed, as they can provide guidance, support, and tools to navigate and overcome negative self-perceptions.

Self-care involves taking care of one's physical, mental, and emotional well-being. Affirmations can play a crucial role in this process. Affirmations are positive statements that can individuals cultivate a sense of self-worth, confidence, and inner peace. They can take various forms, such as daily mantras, positive self-talk, or written affirmations displayed in visible places. Affirmations can be particularly beneficial in a family environment by promoting a positive and supportive atmosphere. When family members practice affirmations, they can boost their self-esteem, create a sense of unity, and foster healthy communication and relationships. By incorporating affirmations into their daily routine, family members can enhance their overall well-being and strengthen their bond with one another.

Examples of Affirmations are listed below:

1. Positive Affirmations: Positive affirmations are that focus on optimistic and encouraging messages to boost self-confidence and promote a positive mindset. Example: "I am capable and worthy of achieving my goals."

2. Gratitude Affirmations: Gratitude affirmations are aimed at expressing appreciation for the blessings and positive aspects of life. Example: "I am thankful for the abundance of love and support in my life3. Self-L Affirmations: Self-love affirmations emphasize self-acceptance, self-care, and building a healthy self-image. Example: "I deserve to treat myself with kindness and compassion."

4. Success Affirmations: Success affirmations help individuals visualize and manifest their goals and achievements. Example: "I attract success and abundance into my life effortlessly."

5. Health Affirmations: Health affirmations focus on promoting physical and mental well-being, healing, and vitality. Example: "My body is strong, resilient, and capable of healing itself."

6. Affirmations for Stress Relief: These affirmations aim to reduce stress and anxiety, promoting relaxation and peace of mind. Example: "I release all tension and embrace a sense of calm and tranquility."

7. Affirmations for Inner Peace: Inner peace affirmations help cultivate a sense of serenity, harmony, and balance within oneself. Example: "I let go of worries and fears, and I embrace peace and harmony within me."

8. Affirmations for Forgiveness: Forgiveness affirmations assist in letting go of past grievances and fostering a sense of forgiveness and compassion. Example: "I forgive myself and others, releasing any resentment and negativity from my heart."

Affirmation and quote for embracing change and finding your inner strength.

Affirmation: "I embrace change and trust in my inner strength to guide me through any challenges that come my way."

Quote: "Strength does not come from physical. It comes from an indomitable will." - Mahatma Gandhi

These different types of affirmations can be tailored to individual needs and preferences to support growth and well-being

By exploring ways to prioritize self-care and promoting a positive body image, we embark on a transformative journey towards embracing our authentic selves, treating ourselves with kindness, and nurturing our physical and mental well-being. This chapter provides practical insights, inspiring ideas, and actionable steps to promote self-love, acceptance, and the creation of a positive body image, ultimately leading to a life filled with confidence, self-empowerment, and overall contentment.

Self-care is a powerful act of self-love and compassion that allows you to recharge, rejuvenate, and nurture your mind, body, and soul. It is a way of honoring yourself and prioritizing your well-being in a world that often demands our constant attention and energy. This is about your long-term health and happiness.

Whether it's indulging in a peaceful morning routine, exercising, meditating, or simply taking time to unwind with a good book, investing in self-care is an investment in yourself. Remember, taking care of yourself is not selfish; it is necessary for your well-being and ability to show up fully in all areas of your life. As the author Audre Lorde once said, "Caring for myself is not self-indulgence, it is self-preservation and is an act of political warfare." So, prioritize self-care to nurture yourself and improve your overall quality of life.

Being an example for your family by prioritizing self-care is a powerful way to inspire others to prioritize their own well-being. By making self-care a priority in your life, you not only benefit yourself, but also set a positive example for your loved ones, encouraging them to prioritize their own well-being and cultivate a healthy work-life balance. Your commitment to self-care can inspire a ripple effect within your family, leading to happier, healthier, and more fulfilling lives for all. Especially your children, it can empower them to prioritize their own well-being, develop self-awareness, and cultivate a positive relationship with themselves. Just by being a role model for self-care, you equip your children with the skills and mindset needed.

Remember, you deserve to care for yourself deeply and unapologetically. Embrace self-care as a revolutionary act of self-empowerment and self-respect. Engaging in activities that nourish your body, mind, and soul, you send a powerful message to your family about the value of taking care of oneself.

- Incorporating relaxation techniques and stress management practices

Amidst the whirlwind of daily life, it becomes increasingly important to carve out moments for relaxation and implement stress management practices. This chapter explores the multitude of techniques and strategies available to help us unwind, reduce stress, and cultivate a sense of calm in our lives.

One powerful tool is the practice of mindfulness, which involves bringing our attention to the present moment and cultivating a non-judgmental awareness of our thoughts, sensations, and emotions. We delve into various mindfulness techniques, such as focused breathing exercises, body scans, and guided meditations. By incorporating these practices into our daily routine, we can cultivate a mental state of calm, improve our ability to handle stressful situations, and foster a greater overall sense of well-being.

Additionally, engaging in physical relaxation techniques can provide immense benefits for our stress levels and overall mental health. Techniques such as progressive muscle relaxation, gentle stretching exercises, and restorative yoga help release physical tension and promote a deep sense of relaxation. We discuss the importance of finding activities that resonate with our individual preferences, allowing us to unwind and rejuvenate our bodies and minds.

Furthermore, exploring stress management practices can lead to healthier coping mechanisms and increased resilience. We delve into strategies such as setting boundaries, managing time effectively, and practicing self-care. Learning to prioritize our needs, delegate tasks, and engage in activities that bring us joy and relaxation can significantly reduce stress levels and promote a more balanced and fulfilling lifestyle.

Incorporating relaxation techniques and stress management practices is an ongoing journey that requires patience and commitment. Through self-reflection, experimentation, and seeking guidance when needed, we can develop a toolkit of practices that work best for us. By making these practices a priority, we can enhance our overall well-being, improve our ability to handle life's challenges, and cultivate a greater sense of peace and tranquility in our lives.

Add a pet, get a dog.

Another way of adding relaxation and stress relief is a family pet. Yes, a family dog is a stress reliever. Adding pets to the family can have a multitude of positive impacts on health and well-being for all members of the household. Firstly, the presence of pets, such as dogs or cats, can provide emotional support and companionship, reducing feelings of loneliness and isolation. Interacting with pets has been shown to decrease stress levels and anxiety, promoting a sense of calm and overall well-being. The responsibility of caring for a pet, including feeding, exercising, and grooming, can also promote a more active lifestyle and routine, leading to improved physical health for both adults and children. Pets can serve as a source of motivation for exercise, especially in the case of dogs that require regular walks. Moreover, the unconditional love and non-judgmental companionship offered by pets can boost self-esteem, increase feelings of happiness, and improve mental health. Studies have shown that owning a pet can lower blood pressure, reduce the risk of heart disease, and even boost immunity. Overall, the presence of pets in the family can create a positive and nurturing environment that can enhance the health and well-being of everyone involved.

What kind of dog should our family consider?

Dog Breeds

1. Labrador Retriever: Labrador Retrievers are known for their friendly and outgoing nature, making them excellent family pets. They are great with children, easy to train, and highly intelligent. Labs are energetic and love to play, making them perfect companions for active families. They also have a gentle temperament, making them a popular choice for households with young children.

2. Golden Retriever: Golden Retrievers are another popular family-friendly breed known for their friendly and loyal disposition. They are gentle, patient, and affectionate dogs that get along well with children and other pets. Golden Retrievers are highly trainable and excel in obedience training. They are also known for their love of outdoor activities and are great companions for families who enjoy spending time outdoors.

3. Beagle: Beagles are small to medium-sized dogs with a friendly and sociable personality, making them great family pets. They are playful, curious, and good with children. Beagles are known for their gentle disposition and are generally good with other pets. They require regular exercise to stay healthy and happy but can adapt well to various living environments.

4. Cavalier King Charles Spaniel: The Cavalier King Charles Spaniel is a small, affectionate breed known for their loving and gentle nature. They are great with children, making them ideal family pets. Cavaliers are social dogs that enjoy human companionship and are easy to train. They are well-suited for apartment living but also enjoy outdoor activities.

5. Poodle: Poodles come in three sizes - standard, miniature, and toy - making them versatile choices for families. They are highly intelligent, trainable, and hypoallergenic, making them suitable for households with allergy concerns. Poodles are friendly, affectionate dogs that enjoy being part of the family. They have a playful nature and thrive on mental stimulation and physical activity.

6. Mixed Breed (Mutt): Mixed-breed dogs can make wonderful family pets and are often available for adoption from shelters and rescue organizations. Mixed-breed dogs come in all shapes and sizes, and each one is unique in terms of temperament and characteristics. By adopting a mixed-breed dog, you are giving a loving companion a forever home while also benefiting from their loyalty, love, and companionship.

In selecting a pet for your family, it's important to consider factors such as energy level, size, temperament, and the amount of time and attention you can dedicate to the pet's care. Additionally, it's recommended to meet the pet in person to ensure compatibility with your family's lifestyle and preferences.

Studies have shown that owning a dog can contribute to an extended life expectancy for humans in various ways. The companionship, love, and emotional support provided by dogs have been linked to lower rates of stress, anxiety, and depression, all of which are known risk factors for various health conditions. Additionally, owning a dog often leads to increased physical activity levels, as dog owners tend to engage in regular walks and exercise routines with their furry companions. This increased physical activity can result in improved cardiovascular health, lower blood pressure, and a reduced risk of obesity. Furthermore, the social interactions that come with being a dog owner can help combat feelings of loneliness and isolation, which are also associated with negative health outcomes. In general, the bond between humans and their canine companions has been shown to have significant benefits for both mental and physical well-being, eventually contributing to a longer, healthier life.

-Family communication and connection

Family communication and connection are vital components of a healthy and functioning family dynamic. Effective communication within a family involves open, honest, and respectful dialogue among its members. This includes not only conveying thoughts and feelings but also actively listening to one another. Strong family connections are built on shared experiences, traditions, and values that create a sense of belonging and unity. Regular communication helps family members understand each other better, resolve conflicts, and support one another through life's challenges. It fosters empathy, and emotional intimacy, strengthening the bonds within the family unit. The importance of family communication and connection cannot be overstated as they contribute to a positive, loving, and supportive environment that promotes individual growth and well-being. By prioritizing communication and connection, families can build stronger relationships and create lasting memories together. Family meetings are an asset to the family.

So, what should you talk about and how to get it going? I will list some examples of topics that families may want to discuss in their family meetings or at any time.

1. Mental health and well-being: Discussing emotions, stress management, and coping strategies as a family can help create a supportive environment where everyone feels comfortable sharing their feelings and seeking help when needed.

2. Healthy lifestyle choices: Conversations about nutrition, exercise, sleep habits, and overall wellness can promote a culture of health within the family and inspire everyone to make positive choices for their physical well-being.

3. Digital well-being: Addressing screen time limits, online safety, and healthy technology habits can help families navigate the digital world responsibly and maintain a healthy balance between technology use and offline activities.

4. Financial literacy: Teaching children about budgeting, saving, investing, and responsible spending can help them develop essential money management skills and create a foundation for financial stability in the future.

5. Diversity and inclusivity: Discussing topics related to diversity, equity, and inclusion can help foster empathy, understanding, and respect for different cultures, identities, and perspectives within the family unit and beyond.

6. Environmental awareness: Conversations about sustainability, recycling, energy conservation, and climate change can raise awareness about environmental issues and inspire family members to adopt eco-friendly practices in their daily lives.

7. Academic and career goals: Encouraging open communication about educational aspirations, career interests, and plans for the future can help family members support each other in achieving their goals and dreams.

8. Conflict resolution: Teaching effective communication skills, problem-solving techniques, and healthy ways to manage disagreements can help family members navigate conflicts constructively and strengthen their relationships.

9. Personal interests and passions: Encouraging discussions about hobbies, creative pursuits, and individual interests can help family members connect with each other, celebrate each other's unique talents, and foster a sense of joy and fulfillment.

10. Current events and social issues: Engaging in conversations about important news topics, social justice issues, and global events can encourage critical thinking, empathy, and a broader understanding of the world around us.

Or and going deeper you can talk about the following example topics.

1. Family values and traditions: Discussing the values, beliefs, and traditions that are important to your family can strengthen bonds and create a sense of shared identity and purpose.

2. Relationship dynamics: Talking openly about communication styles, conflict resolution, and expressing love and appreciation within the family can foster healthier, more fulfilling relationships.

3. Personal boundaries: Setting and respecting personal boundaries within the family can help family members feel safe, respected, and empowered in their interactions with one another.

4. Life goals and aspirations: Sharing dreams, aspirations, and goals for the future can create a supportive environment where family members can encourage and cheer each other on in their endeavors.

5. Sexuality and relationships: Having age-appropriate conversations about sexuality, consent, healthy relationships, and boundaries can help family members navigate these important aspects of life with knowledge and understanding.

6. Emotional support and mental health: Discussing emotions, mental health struggles, and ways to provide support to each other during challenging times can foster a culture of empathy, understanding, and care within the family.

7. Body image and self-esteem: Encouraging positive body image, self-acceptance, and self-love within the family can help create a supportive environment where everyone feels valued and confident in their own skin.

8. End-of-life care and wishes: Having conversations about end-of-life care preferences, funeral arrangements, and estate planning can ensure that family members' wishes are respected and provide peace of mind for everyone involved.

9. Family secrets and past traumas: Creating a safe space for family members to share deeply personal experiences, traumas, and secrets can promote healing, understanding, and forgiveness within the family.

10. Forgiveness and reconciliation: Discussing ways to resolve conflicts, apologize, forgive, and move forward can strengthen familial bonds and create a more harmonious and loving family environment.

Having conversations with the family about both intimate matters and current topics is crucial for fostering strong relationships, promoting understanding, and nurturing a supportive and communicative environment. Discussing intimate matters such as family values, personal boundaries, relationships, and emotional well-being allows family members to connect on a deeper level, build trust, and respect each other's individual needs and perspectives. Likewise, engaging in conversations about current topics such as mental health, diversity, environmental issues, and social justice can broaden family members' perspectives, stimulate critical thinking, and encourage empathy and open-mindedness. Through addressing both intimate and current topics within the family, everyone can feel heard, valued, and supported, leading to stronger bonds, shared values, and a sense of belonging within the family unit.

Family Meetings; A Deeper Connection for Better Health

"Family meetings serve as a time for us to come together and connect on a deeper level".

Family meetings. They allow us to communicate openly, share our joys and struggles, and work together to create a harmonious and supportive environment for all of us."

These meetings help us strengthen our relationships, build trust, and reinforce our family values. They provide a platform for us to address any issues that may arise, resolve conflicts, and celebrate our successes as a family unit."

Research has shown that regular family meetings can have numerous benefits for the health and well-being of family members. By fostering communication, understanding, and empathy, these meetings contribute to improved mental and emotional health, reduced stress levels, and increased feelings of connection and belonging within the family.

Through open dialogue and active listening, family members learn to better understand each other's perspectives, empathize with their struggles, and offer support and encouragement when needed. This strengthens the family bond and creates a sense of cohesion and unity that withstands the challenges of daily life.

Families engaging in a lively discussion about upcoming events, shared goals, and ways to support each other, a sense of collaboration and togetherness can permeate the room. You can brainstorm ideas for fun family activities, planned future vacations, and set mutual goals for personal growth, spiritual and development.

Family meetings. They allow us to communicate openly, share our joys and struggles, and work together to create a harmonious and supportive environment for all of us."

These meetings help us strengthen our relationships, build trust, and reinforce our family values. They provide a platform for us to address any issues that may arise, resolve conflicts, and celebrate our successes as a family unit."

Research has shown that regular family meetings can have numerous benefits for the health and well-being of family members. By fostering communication, understanding, and empathy, these meetings contribute to improved mental and emotional health, reduced stress levels, and increased feelings of connection and belonging within the family.

Through open dialogue and active listening, family members learn to better understand each other's perspectives, empathize with their struggles, and offer support and encouragement when needed. This strengthens the family bond and creates a sense of cohesion and unity that withstands the challenges of daily life.

The impact of these meetings on a family's overall well-being.

"My family and I have these meetings or as we like to call them reasoning sessions. Believe me when I say they are well worth it for the overall health of the family." "Our monthly family meetings not only help us stay connected and communicate effectively but also provide a support system that enhances our resilience and emotional health," for my family. "We learn to appreciate each other's strengths, navigate challenges together, and create a loving and nurturing environment where everyone feels valued and heard."

These family meetings are also beneficial for the small members of the family, and it is wise to include them as well.

Small children in a family can add a unique perspective and energy to family meetings. Their innocence and curiosity can often bring a sense of joy and lightheartedness to discussions that may otherwise be serious or tense. Inclusion of children in family meetings demonstrates that their opinions and thoughts are valued and important, helping to foster a sense of belonging and unity within the family unit. Additionally, young children may provide unexpected insights or solutions to family issues, as they often have a fresh and unbiased view of the world. Their presence can also serve as a reminder to prioritize family relationships and connections, highlighting the importance of spending quality time together and supporting one another. Ultimately, including small children in family meetings can enrich the overall dynamic and enhance the sense of togetherness within the family.

Summary: What Small Children Learn by Having Family Meetings

Engaging small children in family meetings can have a profound impact on their development and well-being. Through participating in these gatherings, young children are given the opportunity to learn valuable life skills, foster positive habits, and strengthen their familial relationships. Here are some key learnings that small children can gain from being involved in family meetings:

1. Communication Skills: By actively participating in discussions, sharing their thoughts, and listening to others, small children can develop essential communication skills. They learn how to express their emotions and ideas, articulate their needs, and engage in dialogue with their family members.

2. Empathy and Understanding: Family meetings teach small children the importance of empathy and understanding towards others' feelings and perspectives. Through actively listening to family members and empathizing with their experiences, children learn to be compassionate and supportive.

3. Problem-Solving Abilities: Family meetings provide small children with the opportunity to engage in problem-solving activities and discussions. By brainstorming solutions, collaborating with family members, and working together to resolve conflicts, children develop critical thinking skills and learn how to navigate challenges effectively.

4. Respect and Consideration: Participating in family meetings instills values of respect, consideration, and inclusivity in small children. They learn to value each family member's opinions, show respect for others' viewpoints, and contribute to a harmonious and cooperative family dynamic.

5. Responsibility and Accountability: Family meetings offer small children a sense of responsibility and accountability as they engage in decision-making processes, set goals, and follow through on family commitments. Children learn the importance of taking ownership of their actions and contributing positively to the family unit.

6. Confidence and Self-Expression: Through active participation in family meetings, small children can build confidence in expressing themselves, sharing their ideas, and speaking in a supportive setting. This fosters a sense of self-assurance and empowerment as children learn to voice their thoughts and opinions.

7. Gratitude and Appreciation: Family meetings cultivate a sense of gratitude and appreciation in small children as they reflect on positive experiences, express thanks for family support, and celebrate shared achievements. Children learn the value of gratitude, kindness, and acknowledging the contributions of others.

8. Family Unity and Bonding: Above all, small children learn the significance of family unity, bonding, and connection through

participating in family meetings. They develop a strong sense of belonging, love, and security within the family unit, fostering lifelong bonds and cherished memories.

By involving small children in family meetings, parents and caregivers provide them with a rich learning experience that extends beyond the meeting room. Small children not only gain valuable skills and values but also internalize the importance of open communication, mutual respect, and shared participation in nurturing a supportive and loving family environment.

Here is an example of a detailed family meeting schedule:

Family Meeting Agenda

Date: Saturday, May 15, 2023

Time: 10:00 AM - 12:00 PM

Location: Family Room

1. Opening (10:00 AM - 10:15 AM)

- Welcome and Introduction

- Review of Meeting Agenda

- Setting Ground Rules (Respect, Listening, One Person Speaks at a Time)

2. Review of Previous Action Items (10:15 AM - 10:30 AM)

- Discuss progress on last meeting's action items

- Determine completion status and next steps

3. Family Updates (10:30 AM - 10:45 AM)

- Each family member shares updates or news from their lives

- Celebrate achievements, share challenges, and offer support

4. Discussion Topics (10:45 AM - 11:30 AM)

- Vacation Planning: Decide on the destination and dates for the next family vacation

- Household Chores Assignment: Review current chore responsibilities and make any necessary adjustments

- Budget Review: Discuss family finances, savings goals, and any upcoming expenses

5. New Business (11:30 AM - 11:45 AM)

- Any additional topics or concerns brought up by family members

- Brainstorm ideas or solutions for any issues raised

6. Action Items and Next Steps (11:45 AM - 12:00 PM)

- Assign specific tasks and responsibilities for each family member

- Set timelines and follow-up plans for completing action items

- Confirm date and time for the next family meeting

7. Closing (12:00 PM)

- Recap of decisions made and action items assigned

- Express gratitude for family members' participation and engagement

- End meeting on a positive note

This example provides a structured framework for conducting a productive and engaging family meeting, ensuring that all members have a chance to contribute and that important family matters are discussed and addressed. You can use or modify the example schedule to fit your unique family and its needs as you like. Family meetings can be yearly and include monthly, weekly, or whenever is best for you and your family.

Seeing the purpose and importance of family meetings, how do families begin to have them?

To start a family meeting, it must be opened the floor for discussion, inviting each family member to share their thoughts, concerns, and dreams. The air should be filled with a sense of openness and respect, creating a safe space for everyone to express themselves freely and without judgment. As the meeting should end with hugs and smiles exchanged, the family will come to know that their commitment to regular family meetings is an investment in their collective happiness and harmony. They will find that it is a testament to the power of intentional communication, shared values, and mutual support in fostering strong and healthy family relationships that will stand the test of time. So, let's break it down now.

Summary: How to Start Having Family Meetings

If you're considering incorporating family meetings into your routine to improve communication, strengthen relationships, and promote well-being, follow these steps to get started:

1. Schedule Regular Meetings: Choose a day and time that works best for your family's schedule and commit to holding regular family meetings. Consistency is key to establishing this valuable tradition.

2. Set the Mood: Create a welcoming and comfortable space for your family meetings. Consider dimming the lights, playing soft music, or lighting candles to create a relaxed and inviting atmosphere.

3. Establish Ground Rules: Encourage respectful communication by setting ground rules for your family meetings. This may include taking turns speaking, actively listening to each other, and refraining from interruptions or judgment.

4. Agenda Planning: Create an agenda for each meeting to keep discussions focused and productive. Include topics such as highs and lows of the week, upcoming events, challenges, and goals.

5. Encourage Participation: Encourage all family members to actively participate in the meetings by sharing their thoughts, feelings, and ideas. Ensure that everyone has been given the opportunity to speak and be heard.

6. Reflect and Evaluate: Take time to reflect on the discussions, decisions made, and progress achieved during each family meeting. Evaluate what worked well and what could be improved for future meetings.

7. Celebrate Achievements: Acknowledge and celebrate achievements, milestones, and positive moments shared during the family meetings. This fosters a sense of gratitude, appreciation, and positivity within the family.

8. Adapt and Evolve: Be open to adapting the format, frequency, and structure of your family meetings based on feedback and changing family dynamics. Flexibility is key to sustaining this beneficial practice over time.

In taking these steps and committing to regular family meetings, you can create a supportive and nurturing environment that promotes communication, connection, and overall well-being within your family. Initiate this tradition with enthusiasm, patience, and a genuine desire to strengthen your family bonds, and watch as your relationships flourish and your family thrives.

Part 2: Mental Well-being

Chapter Three: Cultivating a Positive Mindset

Chapter Three: Cultivating a Positive Mindset

In the journey towards self-improvement and personal growth, one of the most essential and transformative aspects is the cultivation of a positive mindset. A positive mindset is a powerful tool that allows individuals to navigate through life's challenges with resilience, optimism, and a proactive attitude. Developing and maintaining a positive mindset is a continuous practice that requires self-awareness, determination, and a willingness to make positive changes in one's thoughts and behaviors.

At its core, cultivating a positive mindset starts with recognizing and challenging negative thought patterns. Often, we are our own worst critics, constantly dwelling on past failures or worrying about the future. However, by becoming aware of these negative thought cycles, individuals can take steps to replace them with more positive and constructive thoughts. This process involves reframing negative situations, focusing on solutions rather than problems, and practicing gratitude for the blessings and opportunities present in everyday life.

Furthermore, fostering a positive mindset involves surrounding oneself with positivity. This includes cultivating meaningful relationships with like-minded individuals who inspire and support personal growth. By building a strong network of positive influences, individuals can create an environment that reinforces their efforts towards cultivating a positive mindset. Additionally, engaging in activities that bring joy, such as hobbies, exercise, or exploring nature, can strengthen positive emotions and contribute to an overall sense of well-being.

Lastly, maintaining a positive mindset also entails embracing failure and setbacks as opportunities for growth. No one is immune to challenges or mistakes, but individuals with a positive mindset view these experiences as steppingstones towards improvement rather than insurmountable obstacles. They learn from their failures, adapt their approach, and persevere with resilience and determination. Cultivating a positive mindset allows individuals to reframe setbacks as learning opportunities, fostering personal growth, and providing motivation to achieve new levels of success.

In summary, cultivating a positive mindset is an ongoing process that empowers individuals to approach life's challenges with optimism, resilience, and proactive attitudes. By challenging negative thought patterns, surrounding oneself with positivity, and embracing failure as an opportunity for growth, individuals can transform their mindset and unlock their full potential. Ultimately, the development of a positive mindset paves the way for greater happiness, fulfillment, and success in all aspects of life.

- Techniques to reframe negative thoughts and foster a resilient mindset

Reframing negative thoughts is a crucial step in cultivating a resilient mindset that empowers individuals to navigate through life's challenges with determination and positivity. One powerful technique to achieve this is cognitive restructuring, which involves identifying and challenging negative thought patterns and replacing them with more positive and realistic thoughts. By consciously questioning the validity of negative beliefs and replacing them with healthier alternatives, individuals can shift their perspective and cultivate a more resilient mindset.

Another effective technique is practicing self-compassion. Often, negative thoughts stem from self-criticism and unrealistic expectations. By practicing self-kindness and treating oneself with compassion, individuals can reframe negative thoughts and foster a resilient mindset. This involves acknowledging personal flaws and mistakes with understanding and forgiveness, rather than self-judgment and harsh criticism. Cultivating self-compassion allows individuals to view setbacks and failures as opportunities for growth, rather than a reflection of their worth or abilities.

Visualizing success and focusing on positive outcomes is another powerful technique to reframe negative thoughts and foster resilience. By envisioning oneself overcoming challenges and achieving success, individuals can boost their confidence and motivation. Visualization helps individuals see beyond the immediate negative circumstances and visualize a brighter future. It provides a sense of hope and optimism, which fuels the resilience needed to persist in the face of adversity.

Practicing gratitude is yet another effective technique to reframe negative thoughts and foster a resilient mindset. By intentionally focusing on the positive aspects of life and expressing gratitude for them, individuals can shift their attention away from negativity and train their minds to recognize and appreciate the blessings and opportunities present in everyday life. Gratitude cultivates an optimistic outlook and enhances resilience by reminding individuals of the abundance and joy that exists even amidst difficult circumstances.

Reframing negative thoughts and fostering a resilient mindset is essential for individuals to navigate through life's challenges with determination and positivity. Techniques such as cognitive restructuring, practicing self-compassion, visualizing success, and cultivating gratitude can all contribute to this transformative process. By consciously challenging negative thoughts, treating oneself with kindness and understanding, visualizing positive outcomes, and cultivating gratitude, individuals can reframe their perspective and develop a mindset that is resilient, adaptable, and capable of overcoming any obstacle that comes their way.

- Tips for practicing gratitude and mindfulness in daily life

Practicing gratitude and mindfulness can greatly enhance our overall well-being and bring a sense of contentment and peace into our daily lives. Here are some detailed tips to help you incorporate these practices into your routine:

1. Start a gratitude journal: Set aside a few minutes each day to write down three things you are grateful for. This simple practice encourages you to focus on the positive aspects of your life and helps to shift your mindset towards gratitude.

2. Practice mindfulness meditation: Find a quiet and comfortable space where you can sit or lie down. Close your eyes and focus on your breath, bringing your attention to the present moment. Notice the sensations in your body without judgment or attachment. Allow your thoughts to come and go, gently redirecting your focus to your breath whenever your mind wanders. Start with just a few minutes each day and gradually increase the duration.

3. Practice mindful eating: Take the time to fully engage with your meals. Pay attention to the smell, taste, and texture of your food. Chew slowly and savor each bite, being fully present in the experience of eating. This practice not only enhances your enjoyment of food but also helps you cultivate gratitude for the nourishment it provides.

4. Create mindful moments throughout the day: Incorporate short moments of mindfulness into your daily activities. For example, when brushing your teeth, focus on the sensation of the bristles against your teeth and the taste of the toothpaste. When taking a shower, be fully present and notice the feel of the water on your skin. These small moments of mindfulness can help anchor you in the

present moment and develop a sense of appreciation for the simple pleasures of life.

5. Practice gratitude in relationships: Take the time to express your appreciation for the people in your life. Write a heartfelt thank-you note or simply offer a sincere compliment. Engaging in acts of kindness and expressing gratitude not only strengthens your relationships but also cultivates a sense of gratitude within yourself.

6. Nature appreciation: Spend time in nature and allow yourself to fully immerse in its beauty. Observe the colors, sounds, and smells around you. Take deep breaths and feel the connection between yourself and the natural world. Engaging with nature can evoke a sense of gratitude and awe, reminding you of the beauty and abundance that surrounds us.

7. Use visual or verbal reminders: Place reminders in your living or working space to prompt mindfulness and gratitude. It could be a gratitude jar, where you write down things you are grateful for and put them inside. Or you could place inspirational quotes or images that serve as reminders to be present and appreciate the present moment.

Remember, practicing gratitude and mindfulness is a journey, and it takes time and patience to develop these habits. Be kind to yourself and embrace each opportunity to bring more gratitude and mindfulness into your daily life. With practice, these practices can become deeply ingrained and contribute to a more fulfilling and joyful existence.

Chapter Four: Finding Balance in a Busy World

Chapter Four: Finding Balance in a Busy World

In today's fast-paced and tempting world, finding balance is not just a luxury but a necessity. The demands of work, family, social obligations, and personal responsibilities can easily lead to burnout and overwhelm if not properly managed. It is crucial to prioritize self-care and make time for activities that promote balance and well-being. By finding a healthy equilibrium between work and leisure, between activity and rest, and between social connections and personal time, individuals can enhance their overall quality of life and improve their physical, mental, and emotional well-being. Embracing balance allows for greater focus, increased productivity, and a sense of fulfillment that can help navigate the challenges of daily life with grace and resilience.

How do we find balance in a busy world?

Finding balance in a busy world requires intention and mindfulness. One strategy is to prioritize activities that nourish the body, mind, and spirit, such as exercise, meditation, and hobbies that bring joy. Setting boundaries and learning to say no to commitments that do not align with one's values and priorities is also crucial in maintaining balance. Practicing time management and delegating tasks, when necessary, can help to minimize feelings of overwhelm and create space for self-care. Building a support network of friends, family, or professional resources can provide emotional support and encouragement during challenging times. Regularly reassessing one's schedule and commitments to ensure alignment with personal goals and values is key to finding a sustainable balance in the middle of a hectic world.

What are some of the factors keeping you from that needed balance?

In a be here, get there and do this and that world, various factors can hinder individuals from finding balance in their lives. One common obstacle is overcommitment, where individuals take on too many responsibilities or obligations, leaving little time for self-care and relaxation. Perfectionism can also be a barrier to balance, as the constant pursuit of flawlessness can lead to unrealistic expectations and chronic stress. External pressures, such as societal expectations, work demands, and familial responsibilities, can create a sense of overwhelm and prevent individuals from prioritizing their well-being. Technology and constant connectivity can blur the boundaries between work and personal life, making it challenging to disconnect and unwind. Additionally, poor self-care habits, such as lack of exercise, unhealthy eating, and inadequate sleep, can contribute to physical and mental exhaustion, further impeding the ability to find balance. Identifying and addressing these barriers are essential steps toward achieving a more harmonious and fulfilling existence in a fast-paced world.

- Strategies for time management and effective goal setting

Here is an outlined list of strategies for time management and effective goal setting, along with explanations for each strategy:

1. Prioritize tasks: Start your day by listing all the tasks you need to accomplish and prioritize them based on deadlines and importance. This helps you focus on what needs to be done first and reduces the chances of missing deadlines.

2. Set SMART goals: Make sure your goals are Specific, Measurable, Achievable, Relevant, and Time-bound. This helps clarify your objectives and provides a clear roadmap for achieving them.

3. Break down big tasks: Large tasks can be overwhelming, so break them down into smaller, manageable chunks. This makes it easier to tackle each part individually and track your progress more effectively.

4. Use a planner or calendar: Organize your tasks and appointments by using a planner or calendar. This allows you to see your schedule and deadlines immediately, helping you allocate your time efficiently.

5. Time blocking: Allocate specific time blocks for different tasks or activities throughout your day. This helps you maintain focus and prevents distractions by dedicating your attention to one task at a time.

6. Avoid multitasking: While it may seem efficient to juggle multiple tasks simultaneously, studies have shown that multitasking can decrease productivity. Focus on one task at a time to ensure quality output.

7. Set deadlines: Establish deadlines for each task or goal to create a sense of urgency and motivation. Be realistic with your timeline but also hold yourself accountable to meet the deadlines you set.

8. Review and adjust: Regularly review your progress towards your goals and assess if any adjustments or changes are needed. Reflect on what has worked well and what can be improved to optimize your time management strategies.

9. Limit distractions: Identify common distractions in your environment and take steps to minimize them. This might include turning off notifications, setting specific work hours, or working in a quiet space.

10. Practice self-care: Taking care of your physical and mental well-being is essential for effective time management. Make sure to schedule breaks, exercise, and rest to recharge and maintain focus throughout the day.

By incorporating these strategies into your daily routine, you can enhance your time management skills and work towards achieving your goals in a more organized and efficient manner.

Time management and effective goal setting go hand in hand in maximizing productivity and achieving desired outcomes. Below is a detailed example of how to incorporate both into a daily schedule:

Morning Routine:

6:00 am - Wake up and spend 15 minutes for mindfulness meditation to start the day with a clear mind and focus on priorities.

6:15 am - Goal setting: Review long-term and short-term goals, prioritize tasks for the day, and set SMART goals.

6:30 am - Exercise for 30 minutes to boost energy and enhance productivity.

Workday:

8:00 am - Start work by tackling high-priority tasks first to maximize productivity.

10:00 am - Short break to stretch, hydrate, and refocus for the next tasks.

12:00 pm - Lunch break to recharge and rejuvenate.

1:00 pm - Review mid-day progress, adjust schedule if needed, and refocus on remaining tasks.

3:00 pm - Plan for the next day, set priorities, and ensure all tasks are on track.

5:00 pm - End workday and reflect on accomplishments, areas for improvement, and plan for the next day.

Evening Routine:

6:00 pm - Dinner and unwind time to relax and rejuvenate.

7:00 pm - Personal development time: read a book, take an online course, or engage in a hobby.

8:00 pm - Set goals for the next day, review accomplishments, and plan for the week ahead.

9:00 pm - Wind down with a relaxing activity such as meditation, journaling, or light stretching.

10:00 pm - Bedtime routine to ensure 7-8 hours of quality sleep.

Key Points for Effective Time Management and Goal Setting:

1. Prioritize tasks based on importance and urgency to focus on high-impact activities.

2. Break down goals into actionable steps using SMART criteria (Specific, Measurable, Achievable, Relevant, Time-bound).

3. Allocate time blocks for specific tasks and minimize distractions to maintain focus.

4. Review progress regularly and adjust plans as needed to stay on track.

5. Balance work and personal life by scheduling time for self-care and relaxation.

6. Practice self-discipline and consistency in following the schedule to build effective habits.

By merging effective time management strategies and goal-setting techniques into a daily schedule, you can optimize your productivity, achieve your desired outcomes, and maintain a healthy work-life balance.

- Creating healthy boundaries and managing stress

As a writer, I understand the importance of creating healthy boundaries and managing stress to maintain a balanced and productive lifestyle. Setting boundaries allows individuals to establish limits on their time, energy, and relationships, protecting their well-being and preventing burnout. By clearly defining what is acceptable and unacceptable in various aspects of life, such as work, personal relationships, and self-care, individuals can maintain a sense of control and prevent overwhelming. Managing stress is crucial for overall health and mental well-being, as chronic stress can lead to various physical and emotional ailments. By implementing stress management techniques such as mindfulness, exercise, and relaxation techniques, individuals can reduce stress levels and improve their ability to handle challenges effectively. Therefore, prioritizing the creation of healthy boundaries and developing stress management strategies are essential components of leading a fulfilling and sustainable life.

Here's how to create healthy boundaries.

Creating healthy boundaries is essential for maintaining balance and well-being in various aspects of life. To establish healthy boundaries, it is important to first identify your own needs, values, and limits. Understanding what is acceptable and unacceptable to you enables you to communicate your boundaries effectively to others. Be clear and assertive in expressing your boundaries, whether it be in personal relationships, work environments, or social interactions. Setting realistic and firm boundaries helps protect your time, energy, and emotional well-being, promoting self-respect and mutual respect with others. It is crucial to enforce boundaries consistently and be willing to say no, when necessary, even if it may feel uncomfortable. Remember that boundaries are a form of self-care and self-respect and prioritizing them allows you to prioritize your own needs and happiness. Practicing self-awareness, effective communication, and firm boundaries, you can create a healthy and supportive environment that fosters positive relationships and personal growth.

Setting healthy boundaries is essential for maintaining balance, self-care, and positive relationships. Here is a detailed example of how to set healthy boundaries in different areas of life:

1. Personal Boundaries:

- Communicate your needs and limits clearly to others, without feeling guilty or obligated to please everyone.

- Example: If you prefer alone time to recharge, kindly decline social invitations when you need some solitude without overexplaining.

2. Work Boundaries:

- Establish clear work hours, breaks, and expectations with colleagues to prevent burnout and maintain work-life balance.

- Example: Communicate your availability and preferred communication channels to avoid responding to work-related emails or calls during personal time.

3. Social Boundaries:

- Choose relationships that are supportive, respectful, and aligned with your values, and set boundaries when needed to protect your well-being.

- Example: Politely decline invitations or conversations that make you uncomfortable or compromise your values or boundaries.

4. Digital Boundaries:

- Limit screen time, establish tech-free zones, and set boundaries for social media and communication to prioritize real-life connections.

- Example: Implementing a no-phone policy during mealtimes or social gatherings to focus on in-person interactions.

5. Emotional Boundaries:

- Recognize and honor your emotions, express them authentically, and establish boundaries to protect your emotional well-being.

- Example: Clearly communicate your emotional needs and triggers to loved ones and kindly request their support and understanding.

6. Physical Boundaries:

- Respect your body and personal space, set physical boundaries with others, and prioritize safety and comfort.

- Example: Clearly communicate your physical boundaries in intimate relationships and friendships, and assertively enforce them if they are violated.

7. Time Boundaries:

- Prioritize commitments, delegate tasks, and schedule time for self-care, hobbies, and relaxation to prevent overwhelm and burnout.

- Example: Set aside dedicated "me time" on your schedule for self-care activities such as exercise, reading, or hobbies, and honor this time as non-negotiable.

Remember, setting healthy boundaries is an ongoing process that requires self-awareness, assertiveness, and self-compassion. It is fundamental to communicate your boundaries assertively, enforce them consistently, and prioritize your well-being in all aspects of your life.

While discussing boundaries we cannot forget that happy yet dreaded moment when our children become adults and leave to start their new lives. When children become adults and leave the family home, parents often experience a mix of emotions ranging from pride and joy to sadness and loss. This transition can lead to a phenomenon known as empty nest syndrome, where parents may feel a sense of emptiness, loneliness, and a loss of purpose now that their parenting role has shifted significantly." I can admit it was like I was in mourning and seriously felt lost. I was looking through baby and childhood pictures and all. Yet I also felt some pride because they did fly the nest and were soaring."

As parents of adult children, boundaries and relationships undergo a significant transformation, shifting from a more authoritative role to one based on mutual respect, autonomy, and equality. With adult children, it becomes essential to establish clear boundaries that respect their independence and allow them to make their own decisions while still offering support and guidance when needed. Parents may need to navigate a new dynamic where they provide advice and assistance as trusted mentors rather than as direct caregivers.

To cope with empty nest syndrome, it is important for parents to acknowledge their feelings, seek support from friends, family, or a therapist, and focus on self-care and pursuing interests and hobbies that bring them joy and fulfillment. Setting boundaries for empty nest syndrome involves establishing healthy routines, maintaining open communication with adult children, and nurturing other relationships and aspects of life outside of parenting.

Communication becomes key in maintaining healthy relationships, as parents and adult children learn to navigate new roles, expectations, and boundaries. Respect for each other's autonomy, opinions, and life choices becomes paramount, as both parties navigate the complexities of transitioning into a more equal and adult-to-adult relationship. Ultimately, the relationship between parents and adult children evolves into a partnership built on trust, understanding, and mutual respect, creating space for growth, learning, and deepening connections in this new phase of life. By setting boundaries, parents can navigate this period of transition with grace, embrace new opportunities for personal growth and fulfillment, and at the end of the day find a renewed sense of purpose and fulfillment in this new chapter of their lives.

Part 3: Emotional Balance

Chapter Five: Nurturing Emotional Intelligence

Chapter Five: Nurturing Emotional Intelligence

Nurturing emotional intelligence is a vital aspect of personal growth and well-being, allowing individuals to understand and manage their own emotions effectively while also empathizing with the emotions of others. As a result of developing emotional intelligence, individuals can cultivate self-awareness, self-regulation, motivation, empathy, and social skills. This awareness and understanding of emotions enable individuals to navigate through life's challenges with resilience and compassion, fostering stronger relationships and effective communication. Emotional balance plays a crucial role in maintaining mental health and overall wellness, as it allows individuals to cope with stress, conflict, and uncertainty in a healthy manner. By cultivating emotional intelligence and striving for emotional balance, individuals can enhance their ability to make sound decisions, build meaningful connections, and lead a more fulfilling and harmonious life. Prioritizing emotional well-being through mindfulness, self-reflection, and compassionate communication can lead to greater self-acceptance, emotional resilience, and personal growth.

- Understanding emotions and building healthy relationships

Understanding emotions is a fundamental aspect of building healthy relationships, as it allows individuals to communicate effectively, empathize with others, and foster meaningful connections. By developing emotional intelligence and awareness, individuals can recognize and acknowledge their own emotions as well as the emotions of others, leading to greater understanding and harmony in relationships. When individuals are attuned to their own feelings and reactions, they are better equipped to express themselves authentically and respond to others with empathy and sensitivity. This emotional awareness forms the foundation for building trust, respect, and open communication in relationships. Additionally, cultivating a safe and supportive environment where emotions can be expressed and understood without judgment is essential for creating healthy and enriching connections. By prioritizing emotional understanding and communication, individuals can nurture strong, resilient, and fulfilling relationships that promote mutual growth and well-being.

Nurturing emotional intelligence requires attention and practice in various areas of life to develop a deeper understanding and mastery of emotions. Some essential examples of areas where individuals can work on nurturing their emotional intelligence include self-awareness, self-regulation, empathy, social skills, and motivation. Self-awareness involves recognizing and understanding one's own emotions, thoughts, and behaviors, as well as their impact on oneself and others. Self-regulation involves managing and controlling emotions effectively, especially in challenging situations, by practicing techniques like mindfulness and stress management. Empathy entails the ability to understand and empathize with the feelings and perspectives of others, fostering stronger connections and communication. Social skills involve building and maintaining positive relationships, resolving conflicts, and effective teamwork through clear communication and collaboration. Lastly, motivation involves setting goals, persevering in the face of obstacles, and maintaining a positive outlook to achieve personal and professional success. By working on these areas and practicing emotional intelligence skills, individuals can enhance their emotional well-being, interpersonal relationships, and overall success in various aspects of life.

- Tools for managing and expressing emotions in a constructive manner

Managing and expressing emotions in a constructive manner is essential for maintaining mental well-being and nurturing positive relationships. There are various tools and strategies that individuals can utilize to effectively navigate their emotions and communicate them in a healthy way. One powerful tool is mindfulness, which involves being present in the moment and observing one's thoughts and feelings without judgment. By practicing mindfulness, individuals can gain clarity and perspective on their emotions, allowing them to respond thoughtfully rather than react impulsively. Another helpful tool is journaling, where individuals can write down their emotions, thoughts, and experiences as a means of self-reflection and emotional processing. Journaling can help individuals better understand their triggers and patterns of behavior, leading to increased self-awareness and insight. Additionally, seeking support from trusted friends, family members, or mental health professionals can provide a valuable outlet for expressing emotions and receiving guidance and validation. Engaging in physical activities such as exercise, yoga, or meditation can also help individuals release pent-up emotions and reduce stress. By incorporating these tools into their daily routine, individuals can effectively manage their emotions, communicate with them constructively, and cultivate emotional well-being and healthier relationships.

Managing and expressing emotions effectively is crucial for mental and emotional well-being. Here is a detailed example of how to manage and express emotions in a healthy way:

1. Identify Emotions:

- Take time to recognize and label your emotions accurately. Consider using a feelings chart or journaling to track and explore your emotional experiences.

2. Understand Triggers:

- Reflect on what triggers certain emotions and how past experiences or beliefs may influence your emotional responses. This self-awareness can help you better manage your reactions.

3. Emotional Regulation Techniques:

- Practice mindfulness, deep breathing, progressive muscle relaxation, or meditation to calm your mind and body when feeling overwhelmed by emotions.

4. Healthy Coping Strategies:

- Engage in activities that help you decompress and process emotions, such as exercise, creative expression, talking to a therapist, or spending time in nature.

5. Communication:

- Express your feelings assertively and constructively with others, using "I" statements to take ownership of your emotions without blaming or accusing.

6. Setting Boundaries:

- Establish boundaries with others to protect your emotional well-being, communicate your limits, and assertively enforce them when needed.

7. Seek Support:

- Reach out to trusted friends, family members, or mental health professionals for guidance, validation, and support in managing difficult emotions.

Example Scenario:

You feel overwhelmed and anxious about an upcoming work deadline. Instead of bottling up your emotions, you decide to manage and express them in a healthy way:

1. Identify Emotions:

- Recognize that you are feeling anxious and stressed about the deadline.

2. Understand Triggers:

- Reflect on past experiences where deadlines caused similar feelings of anxiety and acknowledge any negative self-talk or perfectionistic tendencies influencing your emotions.

3. Emotional Regulation Techniques:

- Practice deep breathing exercises to calm your nerves and focus on the present moment to prevent spiraling into catastrophic thinking.

4. Healthy Coping Strategies:

- Take a short walk outside to clear your mind, listen to calming music, or engage in a brief mindfulness practice to center yourself before tackling tasks.

5. Communication:

- Reach out to your supervisor or team members to discuss realistic expectations, express your concerns, and request any necessary support or resources to help meet the deadline effectively.

6. Setting Boundaries:

- Communicate your limits regarding additional tasks or responsibilities leading up to the deadline to avoid burnout and maintain a healthy work-life balance.

7. Seek Support:

- Talk to a colleague or friend about your feelings to gain perspective, validation, and emotional support during this challenging time.

With implementing these strategies in managing and expressing emotions, you can cultivate emotional intelligence, resilience, and healthier relationships with yourself and others. Remember to be patient and compassionate with yourself as you navigate your emotional experiences. Keep in mind that everything is and will be okay, and that you are loved and cherished.

Chapter Six: Building Resilience and Overcoming Challenges

Chapter Six: Building Resilience and Overcoming Challenges

Building resilience and overcoming challenges are crucial aspects of personal growth and success in life. Resilience allows individuals to bounce back from adversity, setbacks, and obstacles with strength, adaptability, and determination. By developing resilience, individuals can navigate through life's ups and downs with grace and perseverance, learning from challenges and using them as opportunities for growth and transformation. Resilient individuals are able to manage stress, cope with uncertainty, and overcome obstacles with resilience, enabling them to respond to setbacks with resilience, optimism, and a growth mindset. By cultivating resilience, individuals can enhance their ability to persevere, problem-solve, and thrive in the face of adversity. Overcoming challenges is a key component of resilience, as it requires courage, resilience, and determination to move past obstacles and achieve personal and professional goals. By viewing challenges as opportunities for growth, learning, and resilience-building, individuals can develop the strength and skills needed to overcome setbacks, achieve success, and lead a fulfilling and empowered life.

Bouncing Back from Adversity: The Impact on the Body

Life is full of challenges and obstacles that can test our resilience and strength. Adversity comes in many forms, from unexpected setbacks to major life changes, and how we respond to these challenges can have a significant impact on both our mental and physical well-being. In the face of adversity, the ability to bounce back and overcome difficulties is crucial for maintaining a healthy body and mind.

When faced with adversity, the body goes through a series of physiological responses that can have both positive and negative effects. Stress is a natural response to adversity, triggering the release of hormones such as cortisol and adrenaline that prepare the body for fight or flight. While short-term stress can be beneficial in helping us respond to immediate threats, chronic stress can have a detrimental impact on the body.

Chronic stress has been linked to a variety of negative health outcomes, including increased risk of heart disease, obesity, and other chronic conditions. Prolonged exposure to stress hormones can impair the immune system, disrupt sleep patterns, and lead to inflammation throughout the body. Over time, these effects can take a toll on overall health and well-being.

On the other hand, the ability to bounce back from adversity can have a positive impact on the body. Resilience is the ability to adapt and recover from challenges, setbacks, and trauma, and it plays a key role in promoting physical health and longevity.

In the end, bouncing back from adversity can have a profound impact on the body. While facing challenges is a natural part of life, how we respond to adversity can make a significant difference in our overall health and well-being. By developing resilience and coping strategies, individuals can better manage stress, promote physical health, and thrive in the face of life's difficulties.

Bouncing back from adversity is a powerful and transformative process that can have numerous positive effects on the body.

Bouncing back from adversity is a powerful and transformative process that can have numerous positive effects on the body. Adversity, whether it be physical, emotional, or mental, can take a toll on our health and well-being. However, overcoming challenges and setbacks can lead to a range of physical benefits that can enhance our overall health and resilience.

One of the primary benefits of bouncing back from adversity on the body is increased resilience. When we face and overcome difficult situations, our bodies learn to adapt and become more resilient to stress and adversity. This resilience can help strengthen our immune system, reduce the risk of chronic illnesses, and improve overall physical health.

Moreover, overcoming adversity can also have positive effects on the body in terms of stress relief. Dealing with challenges often leads to increased stress levels, which can have detrimental effects on our physical health. However, when we successfully navigate through tough times, our bodies release feel-good hormones such as endorphins and oxytocin, which can help reduce stress and promote relaxation.

In addition, bouncing back from adversity can boost our self-esteem and confidence, which in turn can have a positive impact on our physical health. When we overcome challenges, we prove to ourselves that we are capable and strong, which can improve our mental outlook and overall well-being. Confidence and self-esteem have been linked to better physical health outcomes, such as lower rates of cardiovascular disease and improved immune function.

Furthermore, the process of overcoming adversity often involves setting goals, making positive changes, and developing healthy coping mechanisms. These actions can lead to improved lifestyle habits, such as regular exercise, balanced diet, and better sleep patterns, all of which contribute to better physical health and well-being.

Overall, the benefits of bouncing back from adversity on the body are numerous and significant. By developing resilience, reducing stress, boosting self-esteem, and fostering healthy habits, overcoming challenges can lead to improved physical health and a greater sense of overall well-being. It is through facing and conquering adversity that we can truly unlock our body's full potential and thrive in the face of life's challenges.

People who are more resilient tend to have lower levels of stress, better immune function, and a reduced risk of developing chronic health conditions.

One key aspect of bouncing back from adversity is developing coping strategies that help manage stress and build resilience. Techniques such as mindfulness meditation, exercise, and social support can help reduce the negative impact of stress on the body and promote overall well-being. Building strong social connections and fostering a sense of purpose and meaning in life can also contribute to resilience and help individuals navigate through difficult times.

Be strong and remember that trouble doesn't always last. Your joy comes in the morning, leaving the past behind. Don't lay or wallow in misery, get up so you can push forward in victory.

- Exploring techniques to bounce back from adversity and develop inner strength

Here is an in-depth guide exploring techniques to bounce back from adversity and develop inner strength:

1. Cultivate a Growth Mindset: Embrace challenges as opportunities for growth and learning rather than viewing them as failures. By maintaining a positive and resilient mindset, you can approach setbacks with optimism and determination.

2. Practice Self-Compassion: Be kind and understanding towards yourself during difficult times. Treat yourself with the same compassion and empathy you would offer a friend facing challenges, acknowledging that setbacks are a natural part of life.

3. Build a Support System: Surround yourself with positive and encouraging individuals who uplift and support you during challenging times. Seek guidance, empathy, and perspective from friends, family, mentors, or support groups to navigate adversity with strength.

4. Develop Coping Strategies: Identify healthy coping mechanisms that work best for you, such as mindfulness, exercise, journaling, or creative pursuits. Engaging in activities that promote relaxation, self-expression, and self-care can help you manage stress and build resilience.

5. Set Realistic Goals: Break down overwhelming challenges into smaller, manageable steps to avoid feeling overwhelmed. By setting realistic and achievable goals, you can make progress gradually and build confidence in your ability to overcome obstacles.

6. Practice Resilience-building Exercises: Engage in practices that promote resilience, such as visualization, gratitude journaling, or positive affirmations. These exercises can help you cultivate inner strength, optimism, and perseverance in the face of adversity.

7. Learn from Setbacks: Reflect on past challenges and setbacks to extract valuable lessons and insights. Understand what worked well, what can be improved, and how you can apply these learnings to future situations to enhance your resilience and problem-solving skills.

8. Focus on Self-Care: Prioritize your physical, emotional, and mental well-being by practicing self-care routines that nourish and rejuvenate you. Establish healthy habits such as proper sleep, nutrition, exercise, and stress management techniques to support your overall resilience.

9. Seek Professional Help: If you find it challenging to cope with adversity on your own, do not hesitate to seek professional help from therapists, counselors, or mental health professionals.

They can offer guidance, support, and tailored strategies to assist you in navigating challenges and building inner strength.

Inserting these techniques into your daily life and mindset, you can cultivate resilience, bounce back from adversity, and develop inner strength to face life's challenges with courage and confidence.

The Thompson family experienced a significant setback when their home was damaged by a severe storm. The house had extensive flooding and structural damage, forcing the family to evacuate and seek temporary shelter. The Thompsons were devastated by the loss of their home and belongings, feeling overwhelmed and uncertain about the future.

Despite the challenges they faced, the Thompson family came together and supported each other during this difficult time. They focused on staying positive and working together to overcome the obstacles ahead. With the help of their community, they were able to find temporary housing and resources to begin the process of rebuilding their home.

As they navigated the process of insurance claims, repairs, and rebuilding, the Thompson family maintained open communication, shared responsibilities, and leaned on each other for emotional support. They found strength in their unity and resilience, knowing that they were in this together and could overcome any adversity as a family.

Over time, the Thompson family successfully restored their home, making improvements to prevent future damage, and creating new memories in the process. Through their experience, they learned the importance of resilience, teamwork, and gratitude for the support of loved ones in times of crisis.

Summary:

In this example, the Thompson family faced a challenging situation when their home was damaged by a storm. Through their unity, communication, and determination, they were able to bounce back from the setback and rebuild their home and their lives. The family's ability to support each other, stay positive, and work together exemplifies the power of resilience and teamwork in overcoming adversity. The Thompson family's story demonstrates that with perseverance, resilience, and the support of loved ones, families can overcome significant setbacks and emerge stronger and more united than before.

- Overcoming self-limiting beliefs and embracing personal growth

Self-limiting beliefs are the negative thoughts and perceptions we hold about ourselves that hinder our personal growth and prevent us from reaching our full potential. These beliefs, often rooted in fear, past experiences, or societal conditioning, create barriers that limit our self-confidence, motivation, and ability to pursue our goals. Overcoming self-limiting beliefs is a transformative journey that involves challenging ingrained thought patterns, building self-awareness, and cultivating a growth mindset to embrace personal growth and unleash our true potential.

Identifying Self-Limiting Beliefs:

The first step in overcoming self-limiting beliefs is to identify and acknowledge them. Reflect on the negative self-talk and recurring doubts that hold you back from pursuing your dreams and exploring new opportunities. Common self-limiting beliefs include thoughts such as "I'm not good enough," "I will never succeed," or "I don't deserve happiness." By becoming aware of these beliefs, you can begin to challenge their validity and understand how they impact your thoughts, emotions, and behaviors.

Challenging Negative Thoughts:

Once you have identified your self-limiting beliefs, it is crucial to challenge them with a critical and compassionate mindset. Question the evidence supporting these beliefs and consider alternative perspectives that empower and uplift you. Replace negative thoughts with positive affirmations and reminders of your strengths, accomplishments, and resilience. By reframing your mindset and focusing on self-compassion, you can gradually weaken the grip of self-limiting beliefs and cultivate a more empowering narrative about yourself.

Cultivating a Growth Mindset:

Embracing personal growth requires adopting a growth mindset, which entails a belief in your ability to learn, evolve, and overcome challenges through effort and perseverance. Shift your focus from fixed limitations to unlimited possibilities by viewing setbacks as opportunities for learning and growth. Embrace challenges, seek feedback, and celebrate progress along your journey of self-discovery and improvement. By cultivating a growth mindset, you can expand your potential, enhance your resilience, and navigate life with courage and optimism.

Setting Meaningful Goals:

To break free from self-limiting beliefs and pursue personal growth, it is essential to set meaningful and achievable goals aligned with your values and aspirations. Define clear objectives that inspire and motivate you to step outside your comfort zone, take calculated risks, and embrace new experiences. Break down larger goals into manageable steps, track your progress, and celebrate small victories along the way. By setting goals that challenge and excite you, you can transform self-limiting beliefs into catalysts for growth and achievement.

Seeking Support and Guidance:

Overcoming self-limiting beliefs and embracing personal growth is a challenging but rewarding journey that can be facilitated by seeking support and guidance from mentors, coaches, or trusted allies. Surround yourself with individuals who believe in your potential, offer encouragement and constructive feedback, and challenge you to exceed your perceived limitations. Engage in personal development workshops, therapy, or self-help resources that provide tools and strategies for building self-confidence, resilience, and self-awareness.

Conclusion:

In conclusion, overcoming self-limiting beliefs and embracing personal growth is a profound process of self-discovery, resilience, and transformation. By identifying and challenging negative thought patterns, cultivating a growth mindset, setting meaningful goals, and seeking support, you can break free from self-imposed limitations and unlock your innate potential. Embrace a mindset of possibility, resilience, and self-compassion as you embark on a journey of personal growth and empowerment, embracing the journey of becoming the best version of yourself.

Part 4: Spiritual Growth

Chapter Seven: Connecting with Your Inner Self

Part 4: Spiritual Growth

Chapter Seven: Connecting with Your Inner Self

Spiritual Growth Habits: Nurturing the Mind, Body, and Soul for Holistic Health

Exploring the Spiritual:

The pursuit of spiritual growth is often seen as a journey of the soul, a quest for deeper meaning and connection with the divine. However, the benefits of spiritual practices extend beyond the realm of the spiritual, impacting our physical health and overall well-being. In this essay, we will explore how cultivating spiritual growth habits can promote a healthy body, fostering a holistic approach to health that nourishes the mind, body, and soul.

The Connection Between Spirituality and Physical Health:

Research has shown that there is a strong connection between spirituality and physical health, with studies indicating that individuals who engage in regular spiritual practices experience a range of health benefits. Spiritual growth habits such as prayer, meditation, and community worship have been associated with lower levels of stress, improved immune function, and a reduced risk of chronic diseases. Additionally, spiritual practices that promote values such as compassion, forgiveness, and gratitude have been linked to greater psychological well-being and resilience in the face of adversity.

Practical Strategies for Promoting a Healthy Body Through Spiritual Growth Habits:

- Prayer: The act of prayer not only strengthens one's spiritual connection with the divine but also has been shown to have physiological benefits such as reducing blood pressure, lowering stress levels, and promoting a sense of calm and relaxation. Regular prayer can serve as a form of mindfulness practice, helping individuals center themselves and manage stress in a healthy way.

- Meditation: Mindfulness meditation, a practice rooted in many spiritual traditions, has been found to have numerous physical health benefits, including reducing inflammation, enhancing immune function, and improving sleep quality. By cultivating a regular meditation practice, individuals can promote a sense of peace, clarity, and well-being that extends to their physical health.

- Community Worship: Engaging in communal worship and participating in religious or spiritual gatherings have been shown to foster a sense of social connection, belonging, and support, which are essential for maintaining good physical health. Studies have indicated that individuals who are part of supportive religious communities tend to have better physical health outcomes and a lower risk of illness.

The Mind-Body-Soul Connection:

Spiritual growth habits not only benefit the physical body but also contribute to the well-being of the mind and soul. The mind-body-soul connection is an integral aspect of holistic health, recognizing the interplay between our thoughts, emotions, spiritual beliefs, and physical health. By nurturing all aspects of our being through spiritual practices, we create a harmonious balance that supports our overall health and vitality.

Wrapping up:

In conclusion, cultivating spiritual growth habits is not only beneficial for the soul but also promotes a healthy body and mind. By engaging in practices such as prayer, meditation, and community worship, individuals can nourish their spiritual well-being while reaping the physical health benefits that accompany these practices. Embracing a holistic approach to health that encompasses the mind, body, and soul allows individuals to experience greater vitality, resilience, and overall well-being. As we continue our journey of spiritual growth, may we remember that nurturing our spiritual selves is not only a path to inner peace and fulfillment but also a way to promote a healthy and vibrant life in all its dimensions.

Connecting with Your Inner Self: A Journey of Self-Discovery and Reflection

In this fast-paced and chaotic world, it's easy to become disconnected from our true selves amidst the noise and distractions of daily life. However, taking the time to connect with our inner self is essential for personal growth, self-awareness, and overall well-being. This journey of self-discovery and reflection can lead to a deeper understanding of who we are, what we value, and what brings us joy and fulfillment.

Connecting with your inner self begins with mindfulness and self-awareness. By tuning into your thoughts, emotions, and physical sensations, you can gain insight into your true feelings and desires. This self-reflection allows you to explore your values, beliefs, and aspirations, helping you align your actions with your authentic self.

One powerful way to connect with your inner self is through practices such as meditation and journaling. Meditation allows you to quiet the chatter of the mind and cultivate a sense of inner peace and clarity. By sitting in stillness and observing your thoughts without judgment, you can gain a deeper understanding of your true nature and cultivate a sense of presence and mindfulness in your daily life.

Journaling is another valuable tool for self-exploration and reflection. By putting your thoughts and feelings on paper, you can create a space for honesty and introspection. Journaling can help you process emotions, gain insight into recurring patterns or themes in your life, and set intentions for personal growth and self-improvement.

Connecting with your inner self also involves listening to your intuition and inner wisdom. Intuition is a powerful guide that can steer you towards decisions that align with your true self and lead to greater fulfillment and happiness. By tuning into your intuition through practices such as meditation and mindfulness, you can learn to trust your inner voice and make choices that are in harmony with your authentic self.

In addition to individual practices, connecting with your inner self can also involve seeking guidance from mentors, therapists, or spiritual teachers who can help facilitate your self-discovery journey. By engaging in conversations and reflections with others who have walked a similar path, you can gain new perspectives, insights, and tools for personal growth and self-exploration.

In conclusion, connecting with your inner self is a transformative journey of self-discovery and reflection that can lead to greater self-awareness, personal growth, and overall well-being. By practicing mindfulness, meditation, journaling, and listening to your intuition, you can cultivate a deeper understanding of who you are and what brings you joy and fulfillment. This journey of self-connection is essential for living a purposeful and authentic life aligned with your true self.

- Exploring different spiritual practices and finding what resonates

Christian spiritual practices play a significant role in deepening one's faith, fostering a closer relationship with God, and nurturing personal growth. These practices are varied and diverse, offering individuals a range of ways to connect with the divine and cultivate spiritual well-being. In this essay, we will explore several Christian spiritual practices and discuss the ways in which they can be used to enhance one's spiritual journey and overall fulfillment.

Prayer:

One of the foundational spiritual practices within Christianity is prayer. Prayer is a direct line of communication with God, allowing individuals to express their hopes, fears, gratitude, and petitions. Through prayer, Christians can develop a sense of intimacy with God, seek guidance and wisdom, and experience a deep sense of peace and comfort. Different forms of prayer, such as intercessory prayer, meditative prayer, and contemplative prayer, offer unique opportunities for individuals to engage with God in ways that resonate with their personal spiritual needs.

Meditation:

Meditation is another powerful spiritual practice that can help individuals quiet their minds, center their hearts, and focus on the presence of God. Christian meditation often involves reflection on scripture, the life of Jesus, or the nature of God's love and grace. By entering a state of inner stillness and receptivity, individuals can cultivate a deeper awareness of God's presence and experience a profound sense of peace and spiritual renewal. Meditation can be practiced individually or in community, providing opportunities for both solitude and shared contemplation.

Fasting:

Fasting is a practice that involves abstaining from food or certain activities for a certain period to draw closer to God, deepen one's spiritual discipline, and cultivate a spirit of self-denial and reliance on God's strength. Fasting can take many forms, such as abstaining from some or all foods, technology, or distractions, and can be practiced individually or as part of a community or church-wide initiative. Through fasting, individuals can experience a heightened sense of spiritual clarity, direction, and dependence on God for sustenance and guidance.

Liturgy and Worship:

Liturgy and corporate worship are essential components of Christian spiritual practice, providing opportunities for individuals to engage with God in community, express their faith through song and prayer, and partake in the sacraments of the Church. Liturgical practices, such as the Eucharist, baptism, and confession, help individuals connect with the larger body of Christ and participate in the timeless traditions of the faith.

Corporate worship offers a sacred space for

individuals to come together as a community of believers, to seek God's presence, and to be transformed by the power of the Holy Spirit.

A deeper look into Spiritual Growth:

Foundations of faith and salvation are central concepts in Christian theology. They form the cornerstone of belief and practice for many Christian denominations. Let me provide you with a detailed summary and list of key points related to these foundational principles:

Foundations of Faith:

1. Belief in God: Central to the Christian faith is the belief in one God who is loving, just, and all-powerful.

2. The Trinity: Christians believe in the doctrine of the Trinity, which states that God exists as three persons - the Father, the Son (Jesus Christ), and the Holy Spirit - in one essence.

3. The Bible: Christians believe that the Bible is the inspired Word of God and serves as the ultimate authority for faith and practice.

4. The Incarnation: Christians believe that Jesus Christ is the Son of God who became human to save humanity from sin.

5. The Atonement: Christians believe that Jesus' sacrificial death on the cross atoned for the sins of humanity and reconciled them with God.

6. The Resurrection: Christians believe in the bodily resurrection of Jesus Christ, which provides hope for eternal life.

7. Salvation by Grace: Christians believe that salvation is a gift from God, received through faith in Jesus Christ, and not based on works or merit.

8. The Church: Christians believe in the importance of the church as the body of Christ, where believers can grow in faith, worship together, and serve others.

9. The Second Coming: Christians believe in the future return of Jesus Christ to establish his kingdom and judge the world.

Foundations of Salvation:

1. Repentance: Recognizing and turning away from sin is essential for receiving salvation.

2. Faith: Trusting in Jesus Christ as Savior and Lord is necessary for salvation.

3. Confession: Acknowledging one's faith in Jesus Christ publicly is a declaration of salvation.

4. Baptism: Baptism symbolizes the washing away of sin and the new life in Christ.

5. Holy Spirit: The Holy Spirit is the guide, helper, and sanctifier of believers, empowering them to live a life pleasing to God.

6. Eternal Life: Salvation offers the promise of eternal life with God in heaven for those who believe in Jesus Christ.

I hope this information helps to deepen your understanding of the foundations of faith and salvation in the Christian tradition. If you have any more questions or need further clarification, feel free to ask a Christian teacher or pastor.

Conclusion:

In conclusion, exploring different Christian spiritual practices can enrich one's spiritual journey, deepen one's relationship with God, and foster personal growth and fulfillment. Whether through prayer, meditation, fasting, liturgy, or worship, individuals can find meaningful ways to connect with Jesus Christ, draw closer to God, and experience the transformative power of the Holy Spirit in their lives. Through engaging in these practices with intentionality, openness, and a desire to grow in faith, individuals can cultivate a vibrant and life-giving spirituality that sustains them on their journey of discipleship and brings them closer to the heart of God.

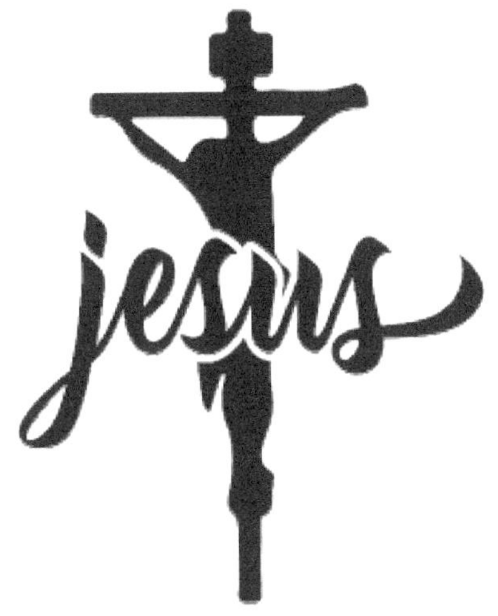

- Cultivating self-awareness and deepening personal values

Introduction:

In a world filled with constant distractions and external influences, the journey towards self-awareness and the deepening of personal values has never been more crucial. By taking the time to introspect, reflect, and engage in intentional practices, individuals can cultivate a deeper understanding of themselves and their core beliefs, leading to a more authentic and fulfilling life. In this essay, we will explore the importance of self-awareness and personal values, as well as practical strategies for nurturing these aspects of our inner lives.

Self-Awareness:

Self-awareness is the foundation upon which personal growth and authenticity are built. It involves the ability to recognize and understand one's own emotions, thoughts, patterns of behavior, and values. Cultivating self-awareness requires a willingness to engage in honest self-reflection, to confront uncomfortable truths about oneself, and to embrace both strengths and weaknesses with compassion and humility. Developing self-awareness, individuals can gain greater clarity about their motivations, desires, and purpose, leading to more intentional decision-making and a sense of inner alignment.

Practical Strategies for Cultivating Self-Awareness:

- Journaling: Keeping a journal allows individuals to record their thoughts, feelings, and experiences, providing a space for introspection and self-expression. Regular journaling can help individuals track patterns, identify triggers, and gain insights into their inner world.

- Mindfulness Practice: Mindfulness involves paying attention to the present moment with openness and curiosity, without judgment. Practicing mindfulness meditation and incorporating mindfulness into daily activities, individuals can become more attuned to their thoughts, emotions, and bodily sensations, fostering a greater sense of self-awareness.

- Seeking Feedback: Soliciting feedback from trusted friends, mentors, or counselors can offer valuable perspectives and insights into one's blind spots and areas for growth. Being open to feedback and willing to learn from others can deepen self-awareness and enhance personal development.

Deepening Personal Values:

Personal values are guiding principles that reflect what is most important to individuals and shape their beliefs, decisions, and actions. Deepening personal values involves clarifying one's core beliefs, identifying priorities, and aligning one's behavior with those values in everyday life. In living in accordance with one's values, individuals can experience a greater sense of integrity, purpose, and fulfillment.

Practical Strategies for Deepening Personal Values:

- Reflect on Core Beliefs: Take time to reflect on what matters most to you, what principles guide your decisions, and what ideals you strive to embody. Clarifying your core values can help you make choices that are aligned with your authentic self.

- Set Intentions: Establish clear intentions based on your values and goals. By setting intentions for how you want to show up in various areas of your life, you can create a framework for living in alignment with your values.

- Practice Ethical Decision-Making: When faced with choices or dilemmas, consider how your values inform your decisions. By consciously aligning your actions with your values, you can cultivate a sense of integrity and authenticity in all aspects of your life.

Conclusion:

In conclusion, cultivating self-awareness and deepening personal values are essential practices for living authentically and meaningfully. By engaging in introspection, self-reflection, and intentional living, individuals can develop a deeper understanding of themselves, clarify their values, and align their actions with their beliefs. In this way, individuals can foster a sense of internal coherence, purpose, and fulfillment that resonates with their truest selves. By embarking on the journey of self-discovery and value clarification, individuals can cultivate a life that is rich in authenticity, integrity, and joy.

Chapter Eight: Living a Purposeful Life

Chapter Eight: Living a Purposeful Life

Living a purposeful life is about aligning one's actions and goals with personal values and beliefs. It involves setting meaningful intentions and striving towards a sense of fulfillment and authenticity. A purposeful life is one in which individuals are driven by a deep sense of passion and meaning, guiding their decisions and actions towards a greater good. It requires introspection, self-awareness, and a willingness to explore one's own strengths and weaknesses. By living a purposeful life, individuals are more likely to experience a sense of inner peace, happiness, and a profound connection to the world around them. Ultimately, living with purpose can lead to a greater sense of fulfillment, impact, and contribution to the greater good.

- Discovering personal passions and aligning actions with values

Discovering personal passions and aligning actions with values is a transformative journey that leads to a more fulfilling and purposeful life. It begins with self-exploration and introspection, as individuals delve deep into their interests, desires, and beliefs to uncover what brings them the most joy and fulfillment. This process often involves trial and error, as individuals experiment with various activities and experiences to determine what truly resonates with their soul. Once personal passions are identified, the next step is to align actions with values. This requires a deep understanding of one's core beliefs and principles, and a commitment to living in accordance with them. When actions are aligned with values, individuals experience a profound sense of authenticity and integrity in all aspects of their lives. This alignment creates a harmonious balance that allows individuals to live with intention and purpose, guiding them towards a life that is rich in meaning and fulfillment. Ultimately, discovering personal passions and aligning actions with values is a powerful journey of self-discovery that can lead to a more authentic, joyful, and purposeful existence.

- Exploring ways to give back and make a positive impact on the world

Exploring ways to give back and make a positive impact on the world is a noble and rewarding endeavor that not only benefits others but also enriches the giver's own life. One effective way to make a positive impact is through volunteering and philanthropy. By donating time, resources, or skills to charitable organizations or causes, individuals can contribute to meaningful projects and initiatives that address important social, environmental, or community issues. Another impactful avenue for creating positive change is through advocacy and raising awareness about important social issues. By speaking out, educating others, and championing causes that are close to their hearts, individuals can help bring about positive change on a larger scale. Additionally, adopting sustainable and environmentally friendly practices in daily life can also make a positive impact on the world by reducing one's carbon footprint and promoting a healthier planet for future generations. Overall, exploring ways to give back and make a positive impact on the world requires dedication, compassion, and a willingness to act, but the rewards of knowing that one has made a difference in the lives of others and the world at large are immeasurable.

Living with a purpose, discovering personal passions, and finding ways to give back to the community can have a profound impact on both the individual and the world around them. Let me provide you with a detailed example to illustrate this concept:

Example: Jane's Journey to Making a Positive Impact

Jane is a young professional who has always had a strong desire to make a difference in her community. Through self-reflection and introspection, she realized that her passion lies in empowering underprivileged youth through education and mentorship. Jane decides to take intentional steps to live with purpose and use her personal passions to make a positive impact:

1. Discovering Personal Passions:

Jane reflects on her own life experiences and realizes that education played a crucial role in shaping her future. She is passionate about ensuring that every child has access to quality education and opportunities for growth. This realization ignites a fire within her to take action and make a difference in the lives of young people.

2. Setting Meaningful Goals:

Jane establishes clear, achievable goals to align with her passion. She aims to volunteer at local schools, provide mentorship to at-risk youth, and advocate for educational opportunities for underprivileged communities. By setting these goals, Jane creates a roadmap for how she can contribute positively to her community.

3. Taking Action:

Jane actively seeks out opportunities to volunteer at schools, participate in mentorship programs, and collaborate with local organizations that share her passion for education and youth empowerment. She uses her skills and resources to impact the lives of students and support their academic and personal growth.

4. Creating Lasting Impact:

Over time, Jane's efforts begin to make a significant impact in her community. She witnesses the positive changes in the lives of the students she mentors, sees academic improvements, and fosters a sense of hope and possibility among disadvantaged youth. By staying committed to her purpose and passions, Jane creates a ripple effect of change that extends beyond herself.

5. Inspiring Others:

Jane's dedication and impact inspire others in her community to get involved and make a difference. Through her example, she motivates her peers, colleagues, and friends to discover their own passions and find unique ways to give back. Together, they form a network of individuals dedicated to creating positive change.

In this example, Jane's journey exemplifies how living with a purpose, discovering personal passions, and giving back to the community can lead to making a meaningful and lasting impact. By following her heart, setting goals, acting, and inspiring others, Jane not only transforms the lives of those she serves but also cultivates a sense of purpose and fulfillment in her own life.

Or

Let me provide you with another example of someone living with a purpose, discovering personal passions, and finding ways to give back to the community to make a positive impact.

Example: Mark's Journey to Making a Positive Impact

Mark is a middle-aged professional who has always felt a deep connection to nature and wildlife. He has a passion for environmental conservation and a desire to protect natural habitats for future generations. Through introspection and self-discovery, Mark realizes that he wants to live a purposeful life by making a positive impact on the environment and the community.

1. Discovering Personal Passions:

Mark reflects on his childhood spent exploring the outdoors, camping, and observing wildlife. He realizes that his love for nature has been a constant source of joy and inspiration in his life. Mark understands that preserving the environment aligns with his core values and brings him a sense of fulfillment.

2. Setting Meaningful Goals:

Mark decides to set specific goals that will allow him to leverage his passion for environmental conservation. He aims to volunteer at local conservation organizations, participate in clean-up initiatives, and educate others about the importance of protecting the environment. By establishing these goals, Mark creates a roadmap for how he can contribute to his community and protect the natural world.

3. Taking Action:

Mark proactively seeks out opportunities to get involved in environmental conservation efforts. He volunteers at a local nature reserve to assist with habitat restoration projects, organizes community clean-up events along a nearby river, and gives educational presentations at local schools about the importance of biodiversity and sustainability. Mark is dedicated to taking tangible actions that align with his values and passions.

4. Creating Lasting Impact:

Over time, Mark's dedication to environmental conservation begins to make a significant impact in his community. He sees positive changes in the local ecosystem, witnesses increased awareness about environmental issues, and fosters a sense of stewardship among community members. By staying committed to his purpose, Mark leaves a long-lasting legacy of conservation and sustainability in his area.

5. Inspiring Others:

Mark's passion and actions inspire others in his community to act and engage in environmental conservation efforts. His enthusiasm for nature and commitment to making a difference motivates his friends, neighbors, and colleagues to join him in protecting the environment. Together, they form a strong network of individuals dedicated to preserving the natural world.

In this example, Mark's journey exemplifies how living with a purpose, discovering personal passions, and giving back to the community can lead to making a positive impact on the environment and society. By following his passion for environmental conservation, setting meaningful goals, by acting, and inspiring others, Mark not only contributes to a healthier planet but also enriches his own life with purpose and fulfillment.

I hope this example illustrates the transformative power of living with a purpose and making a positive impact on the community. If you have any more questions or need further clarification, feel free to ask anyone else who may volunteer their time or has a connection with a community organization and or runs one.

As an individual living with purpose is about finding meaning in your daily actions, aligning your values with your goals, and contributing positively to the world around you. When you live with intention, you cultivate a sense of fulfillment, direction, and impact that extends beyond your individual existence. Discovering your passion for the community allows you to connect with others, create positive change, and foster a sense of belonging and unity with those around you. Families play a crucial role in fostering a sense of purpose and community passion. By discussing and identifying shared values, goals, and causes that resonate with the family members, they can collectively work towards creating a more compassionate and thriving community. Engaging in meaningful conversations and activities that align with their collective values strengthens familial bonds and fosters a sense of togetherness. In conclusion, by embracing a purposeful life and cultivating a passion for the community, individuals and families have the power to create a more compassionate, connected, and resilient society. Through self-reflection, shared values, community engagement, and passion-driven actions, they can make a lasting impact that transcends generations and fosters a sense of unity and common purpose. Together, let us inspire one another to live with intention, compassion, and a deep commitment to building a better world for all.

A part of living a purposeful life includes a unified family. It is important to understand the dynamics of mutual respect and trust within the family; even the lack of it and how to rebuild it.

Mutual respect and trust

Understanding what causes the breakdown of mutual respect and trust in the family.

There are several common issues that can lead to families losing mutual respect and trust within their relationships. Communication breakdowns, such as lack of effective listening or misunderstandings, can create barriers to open dialogue and understanding among family members. Conflicts and unresolved disagreements, if not addressed in a constructive manner, can erode trust and respect over time. Issues related to power dynamics, favoritism, or lack of equal treatment among family members can also contribute to feelings of inequality and resentment, further damaging trust and respect. Additionally, breaches of trust, such as dishonesty, betrayal, or broken promises, can severely impact the foundation of respect and trust within the family. Stress, financial struggles, and external pressures can also strain familial relationships and lead to a breakdown in mutual respect and trust. Recognizing and addressing these underlying problems is essential to rebuilding and strengthening the bonds of respect and trust within the family unit. Efforts to address these issues with empathy, open communication, and a commitment to understanding and supporting one another can help restore trust and respect within the family.

What is mutual respect and trust?

Mutual respect and trust between family members are essential components of a healthy and harmonious family dynamic. Respect forms the foundation of positive interactions and relationships within a family, fostering a sense of understanding, acceptance, and appreciation for each member's individuality and contributions. When family members treat each other with respect, they create a supportive and nurturing environment where everyone feels valued and heard. Trust, on the other hand, is built on honesty, reliability, and integrity, and serves as the glue that holds a family together. Trust enables family members to rely on each other, communicate openly, and feel secure in sharing their thoughts, feelings, and challenges. By cultivating mutual respect and trust, families can strengthen their bonds, resolve conflicts constructively, and navigate life's ups and downs with a sense of unity and resilience. Ultimately, fostering mutual respect and trust within a family cultivates a positive and supportive atmosphere that promotes overall well-being and happiness for all members.

How to fix it if we don't have it.

To address the issue of not having mutual respect and trust in a family, it is crucial to initiate open and honest communication among all family members. Encouraging dialogue and active listening can help identify underlying issues, concerns, and misunderstandings that may be impacting trust and respect within the family unit.

Establishing clear boundaries and expectations, along with promoting empathy and understanding, can also foster a culture of mutual respect. Family members should be encouraged to demonstrate trustworthiness through consistent actions and behaviors that align with shared values and commitments. Additionally, engaging in regular family activities and quality time together can strengthen familial bonds and create opportunities for building trust and respect. Seeking the assistance of a family therapist or counselor may also be beneficial in addressing deeper-rooted issues and facilitating constructive communication and problem-solving strategies within the family. By proactively addressing these areas, families can work towards rebuilding mutual respect and trust, ultimately promoting a harmonious and supportive family environment.

To address the lack of mutual respect and trust in a family, it is important to take proactive steps to rebuild and strengthen these essential components of a healthy family dynamic. Here are some strategies to help fix the problem:

1. Communication: Encourage open and honest communication within the family. Create a safe space where each family member feels comfortable expressing their thoughts, concerns, and emotions. Listen actively and validate each other's perspectives to foster understanding and empathy.

2. Establish Boundaries: Clearly define boundaries and expectations within the family to promote respect for individual differences and personal space. Encourage mutual consideration and establish rules that respect each family member's rights and autonomy.

3. Practice Empathy: Empathy is key to cultivating understanding and compassion within the family. Encourage family members to put

themselves in each other's shoes, acknowledge each other's feelings, and show empathy in times of conflict or difficulty.

4. Build Trust Through Actions: Trust is built over time through consistent actions that demonstrate reliability, accountability, and integrity. Encourage family members to follow through on their commitments, be honest and transparent, and demonstrate trustworthiness in their interactions.

5. Foster Positive Interactions: Create opportunities for family bonding and quality time together. Engage in activities that promote mutual respect and trust, such as sharing meals, going on outings, or participating in group activities that encourage cooperation and collaboration.

6. Seek Professional Help: If the lack of mutual respect and trust within the family is deeply rooted or challenging to address on your own, consider seeking the help of a family therapist or counselor. A trained professional can provide guidance, support, and strategies to facilitate communication, rebuild trust, and strengthen relationships within the family.

Thru implementing these strategies and actively working towards fostering mutual respect and trust, families can overcome challenges, strengthen their bonds, and create a supportive and harmonious environment where all members feel valued and understood.

A unified family

A unified family, where members work together, support each other, and communicate effectively, is essential for fostering a healthy and harmonious family environment. When family members are unified, they create a strong support system that offers emotional, mental, and physical well-being. Unity within the family encourages cooperation, collaboration, and mutual respect, leading to stronger bonds and a sense of belonging for each member. Unified families are better equipped to navigate challenges, handle conflicts constructively, and celebrate successes together. By promoting unity, families can enhance communication, build trust, and create a shared sense of purpose and identity that strengthens familial relationships and promotes overall health and happiness. A unified family not only provides a sense of security and belonging for each member but also fosters a positive and nurturing environment that contributes to the well-being and resilience of the entire family unit.

Without a unified family there is no mutual respect and trust, which destroys the health of the family make-up and the essence of its legacy for generations to come. In the end breeding destructive generational curses. Let's break the cycle and strongholds that plague the family for a healthy and unified connection between members. There are principles of a healthy lifestyle that can help guide the family in its journey to the desired lifestyle.

Principles of a Healthy Family Lifestyle:

1. Communication: Open and honest communication is essential in a healthy family lifestyle. It helps family members express their thoughts, feelings, and needs effectively.

2. Quality Time Together: Spending quality time together as a family, such as eating meals together, playing games, or engaging in activities, strengthens bonds and fosters positive relationships.

3. Healthy Eating Habits: Encouraging nutritious meals and snacks, as well as practicing portion control, can contribute to overall health and well-being for every family member.

4. Regular Physical Activity: Staying active as a family through activities like walking, biking, or playing sports promotes physical fitness and overall health.

5. Emotional Support: Providing emotional support, understanding, and encouragement to one another helps create a positive and nurturing environment within the family.

6. Boundaries and Respect: Establishing boundaries and showing respect for each other's feelings, opinions, and personal space is crucial for maintaining a harmonious family dynamic.

7. Positive Reinforcement: Offering praise, recognition, and positive reinforcement for achievements and efforts helps build confidence and self-esteem within the family.

How to Maintain a Healthy Family Lifestyle:

1. Lead by Example: Parents or guardians should model healthy behaviors and habits for their children to follow.

2. Schedule Family Time: Set aside dedicated time for family activities, meals, or outings to strengthen your family bond.

3. Meal Planning: Plan and prepare balanced meals together as a family, incorporating a variety of nutritious foods.

4. Stay Active Together: Incorporate physical activities that everyone enjoys, such as going for walks, swimming, or playing sports.

5. Communication: Encourage open and honest communication within the family to address concerns, solve problems, and strengthen relationships.

6. Set Goals: Establish health and wellness goals as a family and work together to achieve them, motivating each other along the way.

7. Celebrate Achievements: Recognize and celebrate each other's accomplishments, whether big or small, to reinforce positive behavior and maintain a supportive environment.

By using these principles and maintaining healthy habits, you can help promote a positive and fulfilling family lifestyle.

In the next section I will bring awareness to some of the possible illnesses that can affect your family. Awareness plays a vital role in promoting education, understanding, and preparedness for various issues that affect individuals and families. Also, information on CPR, how to perform it in an emergency along with first aid kits, what goes into one and its importance.

Every household should have a first aid kit as it serves as a crucial resource for handling minor injuries and medical emergencies. Having a well-stocked first aid kit readily available allows for immediate response and treatment of common injuries such as cuts, burns, bruises, and sprains. In situations where professional medical help may be delayed, a first aid kit can make a significant difference in reducing the severity of an injury or preventing complications. Additionally, a first aid kit provides a sense of security and preparedness for unexpected incidents that can occur at any time. By having essential medical supplies and tools on hand, households can effectively manage minor health issues and provide timely care to family members or guests in need. Overall, having a first aid kit promotes safety, readiness, and the ability to respond effectively in times of need, making it an essential item for every household.

Having a first aid kit easily accessible in the home can help provide immediate care and potentially prevent more serious medical complications.

A well-equipped first aid kit should contain a variety of essential items to handle minor injuries and emergencies. Here is a detailed description list of the various items typically found in a first aid kit:

1. Adhesive bandages: These come in various sizes and are used to cover and protect small cuts and wounds.

2. Sterile gauze pads: These are used for cleaning and covering larger wounds to promote healing.

3. Adhesive tape: Used to secure dressings and bandages in place.

4. Antiseptic wipes or solution: Used to clean and disinfect wounds to prevent infection.

5. Tweezers: Essential for removing splinters, debris, or foreign objects from the skin.

6. Scissors: Used for cutting bandages, clothing, or other materials in first aid situations.

7. Disposable gloves: Protect the caregiver from exposure to bodily fluids and contaminants.

8. Instant cold packs: Help reduce swelling and inflammation in case of sprains or strains.

9. CPR face shield: Provides a barrier when performing mouth-to-mouth resuscitation.

10. First aid manual: Offers guidance and instructions on how to respond to different medical emergencies effectively.

Having these items in a first aid kit ensures that you are prepared to provide timely and appropriate care for minor injuries and medical emergencies that may arise at home or while on the go. It is a tool that comes in handy with children in the home, it can reduce the number of emergency room visits that can be handled at home, which can save you some money and time.

Common illnesses that can affect individuals include colds and flu, which are caused by viruses and spread easily within households. It is important for families to practice good hygiene, such as frequent handwashing, to prevent the spread of these illnesses. Other conditions like allergies, asthma, and diabetes can also impact family members' quality of life and require proper management and treatment. Mental health disorders, such as anxiety and depression, are crucial to recognize and address within the family unit to ensure emotional well-being. Additionally, understanding chronic conditions like heart disease, cancer, and hypertension is essential for prevention, early detection, and proper management. By educating yourselves about various illnesses and their symptoms, families can take proactive steps to promote health, prevent illnesses, and seek appropriate medical care when needed.

What does CPR stand for?

Cardiopulmonary resuscitation (CPR) is a life-saving technique used in emergencies when someone's breathing or heartbeat has stopped.

Performing CPR

Performing CPR can help maintain blood circulation and oxygenation to vital organs until professional medical help arrives. Here is a detailed explanation of how to perform CPR:

1. Assess the Situation: Check the scene for any potential hazards before approaching the person needing assistance. Ensure your own safety first.

2. Check Responsiveness: Tap the person on the shoulder and shout their name to see if they respond. If there is no response, the person may be unresponsive and in need of CPR.

3. Call for Help: If there is someone else present, instruct them to call emergency services (911) immediately. If you are alone, perform CPR for about 2 minutes before taking a break to call for help.

4. Check Breathing: Tilt the person's head back slightly and check for signs of normal breathing (look for chest rise and fall, listen for breath sounds, and feel for breath on your cheek). If the person is not breathing or only gasping, start CPR.

5. Perform Chest Compressions:

- Place the heel of one hand on the center of the person's chest (between the nipples) and put the other hand on top.

- Lean over the person, keeping your arms straight, and push down firmly at least 2 inches in depth at a rate of 100-120 compressions per minute.

6. Give Rescue Breaths:

- After 30 compressions, tilt the person's head back and lift their chin to open the airway.

- Pinch the person's nose closed and create a tight seal over their mouth with yours.

- Give two rescue breaths, each lasting about one second, and watch for chest rise.

7. Continue CPR: Repeat cycles of 30 compressions and 2 breaths until help arrives or the person starts breathing on their own.

What to expect during CPR:

- Fatigue: Performing CPR can be physically demanding, and you may tire quickly. Rotate with another rescuer, if possible, to maintain effective compressions.

- Emotional Impact: Providing CPR can be stressful and emotionally challenging. It's essential to remain focused on the task at hand and remember that you are helping to save a life.

- Professional Help: Emergency medical services will take over once they arrive. Provide them with information about what has been done so far and be prepared to assist as needed.

Remember that receiving CPR promptly can significantly increase a person's chances of survival in a cardiac arrest emergency. Training in CPR techniques can help you feel more prepared and confident to act in such situations.

What are some illnesses that may require CPR?

Some common illnesses or situations where CPR may be necessary include:

1. Cardiac Arrest: This is the most common scenario where CPR is required. Cardiac arrest occurs when the heart suddenly stops beating effectively, leading to a lack of blood flow to vital organs. Causes can include heart attacks, arrhythmias, drowning, or severe trauma.

2. Choking: When a person's airway is blocked by a foreign object, such as food or a small toy, it can lead to choking and obstructed breathing. If the obstruction is not relieved promptly, it can result in loss of consciousness and the need for CPR.

3. Drowning: Submersion in water can cause a lack of oxygen to the brain, leading to respiratory distress or cardiac arrest. CPR is often necessary to provide oxygen to the person's body until medical help arrives.

4. Drug Overdose: Certain medications or recreational drugs can lead to respiratory depression or cardiac arrest. Administering CPR may be required to maintain circulation and oxygenation until the effects of the drugs wear off or medical assistance is available.

5. Severe Allergic Reactions: Anaphylaxis, a severe allergic reaction, can cause a sudden drop in blood pressure and difficulty breathing. In extreme cases, it can lead to cardiac arrest, requiring immediate CPR intervention.

6. Sudden Trauma: Severe accidents, injuries, or trauma to the chest can lead to cardiac arrest or respiratory failure, necessitating the initiation of CPR to support vital functions until professional medical help arrives.

7. Heart Attack: A heart attack occurs when blood flows to a part of the heart is blocked, leading to damage to heart muscle tissue. In some cases, a heart attack can progress to cardiac arrest, requiring CPR to maintain blood circulation.

It is important to note that these are just a few examples of situations where CPR may be necessary in an emergency. Being aware of potential risks, understanding the signs of distress, and being prepared to act fast with CPR training can greatly increase the chances of saving a life in a critical situation.

There are other illnesses to be aware of as well, and knowing is truly half the battle. It can be difficult to not know or understand what to do about something you're unaware of or look and feel lost during a situation. No one likes to appear incapable of helping a loved one in front of the family.

Something for families to be aware of is the (HCV) Hepatitis C virus.

Getting tested for hepatitis C is important for you and your family due to several reasons. Hepatitis C is a serious viral infection that can cause liver damage, cirrhosis, and even liver cancer if left untreated. Many individuals with hepatitis C do not experience any symptoms initially, making it crucial to get tested to detect the infection early. By getting tested, you can receive appropriate medical care and treatment to manage the infection, prevent complications, and protect your overall health. Furthermore, by knowing your hepatitis C status, you can take necessary precautions to prevent spreading the virus to your family members or loved ones. Regular testing for hepatitis C is recommended for individuals at higher risk, such as those who have a history of injection drug use, received blood transfusions before 1992, or have engaged in high-risk behaviors. It is essential for both you and your family to prioritize getting tested for hepatitis C to safeguard your health and well-being.

What is Hepatitis C?

Hepatitis C is a viral infection that primarily affects the liver, caused by the hepatitis C virus (HCV). The virus is typically spread through contact with contaminated blood, often through sharing needles or equipment for injecting drugs, receiving a blood transfusion before 1992, or having unprotected sex with an infected individual. Hepatitis C can also be transmitted from mother to baby during childbirth. The infection can lead to both acute and chronic forms of hepatitis, with chronic infection being more common and potentially causing serious liver damage over time. Many individuals with hepatitis C may not experience any symptoms initially, but over time, they may develop fatigue, abdominal pain, jaundice, and other signs of liver inflammation. Hepatitis C is a major global health concern, affecting millions of people worldwide. Early detection through testing, followed by appropriate medical treatment and management, is crucial in preventing complications and preserving liver health.

Hepatitis C: Symptoms, Effects and Treatment

Hepatitis C can present with a wide range of symptoms, although many individuals may not experience any symptoms at all. When symptoms do occur, they can vary in severity and may include fatigue, flu-like symptoms, abdominal pain, loss of appetite, nausea, muscle and joint pain, and dark urine. Some people with hepatitis C may also develop jaundice, where their skin and eyes turn yellow. Chronic hepatitis C infection can lead to more serious complications such as liver cirrhosis, liver failure, and an increased risk of liver cancer. Fortunately, there are effective treatments available for hepatitis C that can help manage the infection and prevent long-term liver damage. The standard treatment for hepatitis C used to involve interferon and ribavirin, but these older treatments had significant side effects and limited effectiveness. Nowadays, direct-acting antiviral medications have revolutionized the treatment of hepatitis C by offering high cure rates with fewer side effects. These newer medications target specific steps in the viral replication process, effectively clearing the virus from the body. With early detection, proper medical care, and adherence to treatment, individuals with hepatitis C can achieve a cure, prevent complications, and preserve their liver health. It is important for anyone at risk of hepatitis C or experiencing symptoms to seek medical advice for testing and appropriate management. It is essential for both you and your family to prioritize getting tested for hepatitis C to safeguard your health and well-being.

Having advance directives

What are they and what are they for?

Having advance directives, such as living wills, medical power of attorney, and other forms, is crucial for families to ensure their wishes are known and respected in the event of nonverbal emergencies or incapacitation. These legal documents provide guidance to healthcare providers and family members about medical treatment preferences and decision-making authority when an individual is unable to communicate their own wishes. Here are some key reasons why families should have these essential documents in place:

1. Ensuring Personal Wishes are Respected: Advance directives allow individuals to document their preferences for end-of-life care, including decisions about life-sustaining treatment, resuscitation, organ donation, and more. Having a living will ensures that healthcare providers and family members understand and honor the individual's wishes, even when they cannot speak for themselves.

2. Designating a Healthcare Proxy: A medical power of attorney document allows individuals to appoint a trusted person as their healthcare proxy or agent to make medical decisions on their behalf if they are incapacitated. This ensures that someone who knows the individual's values and preferences can advocate for their care when they are unable to do so.

3. Avoiding Family Conflict: Having clear and legally binding instructions in the form of advance directives can help prevent disagreements among family members over medical decisions. By outlining preferences in advance, families can reduce the likelihood of conflict and uncertainty during stressful situations.

4. Providing Peace of Mind: Knowing that one's healthcare preferences and decisions are documented and legally recognized can provide peace of mind for both the individual and their loved ones. Advance directives alleviate the burden of decision-making during a medical crisis and ensure that care aligns with the individual's wishes.

5. Facilitating Communication with Healthcare Providers: Advance directives serve as a valuable communication tool for healthcare providers, ensuring that they understand the individual's wishes and can provide appropriate care based on those preferences. This can lead to more effective and compassionate medical decision-making in emergency situations.

6. Preparing for Unexpected Events: Medical emergencies or sudden incapacitation can occur at any time, making it essential to have advance directives in place before such situations arise. Being proactive in creating these documents ensures that one's wishes are known and respected when immediate medical decisions are required.

In summary, having living wills, medical power of attorney, and other advance directives is essential for families to navigate nonverbal emergencies and ensure that medical decisions align with individual preferences and values. Discussing these forms with loved ones and healthcare providers can help facilitate important conversations about end-of-life care and provide clarity and guidance during challenging times. These documents can and will be a great help for your family in the event of such situations. Be prepared so you don't have to rush at the last minute.

Life insurance

What is it all about and is it important?

Life insurance is a financial product that provides a lump-sum payment, known as a death benefit, to beneficiaries upon the insured person's death. It serves as a financial safety net for families by helping to replace lost income, cover outstanding debts, pay for final expenses, and maintain their standard of living in the absence of the primary breadwinner. There are several types of life insurance policies, including term life insurance, whole life insurance, and universal life insurance, each offering different features and benefits.

Here are the key differences in life insurance policies:

1. Term Life Insurance:

- Coverage for a specific period, such as 10, 20, or 30 years.

- Typically, lower premiums compared to permanent life insurance.

- Provides a death benefit if the insured dies during the term of the policy.

- Does not build cash value.

- Ideal for those with temporary financial obligations, such as mortgages or children's education.

2. Whole Life Insurance:

- Provides coverage for the insured's entire life, if premiums are paid.

- Builds cash value over time that can be borrowed against or withdrawn.

- Premiums are generally higher than term life insurance.

- Offers guaranteed death benefit and cash value growth.

3. Universal Life Insurance:

- Offers flexibility in premium payments and death benefits.

- Allows policyholders to adjust coverage levels and premiums over time.

- Builds cash value that earns interest based on market performance.

- Provides permanent coverage and a death benefit.

Now, let's discuss the importance of having life insurance for your family:

1. Financial Protection: Life insurance provides financial security for your family in the event of your death. The death benefit can help cover immediate expenses, such as funeral costs, outstanding debts, and ongoing living expenses.

2. Income Replacement: If you are the primary breadwinner in your family, life insurance can replace lost income and help support your loved ones' financial needs, such as mortgage payments, childcare, and education expenses.

3. Debt Repayment: Life insurance can help settle outstanding debts, such as loans, mortgages, and credit card balances, preventing financial strain on your family members after your passing.

4. Estate Planning: Life insurance proceeds can be used to cover estate taxes, probate costs, and other financial obligations, ensuring a smooth transfer of assets to your beneficiaries.

5. Peace of Mind: Knowing that your loved ones will be financially protected and provided for in your absence can offer peace of mind and alleviate concerns about their future well-being.

6. Legacy Building: Life insurance can be used to leave a financial legacy for your family, supporting their long-term goals and aspirations even after you are gone.

In conclusion, having life insurance is a vital component of comprehensive financial planning, especially for those with dependents or financial obligations. It offers peace of mind, financial protection, and legacy planning benefits for your family, ensuring their continued well-being and stability in the face of unforeseen circumstances. Which is a part of financial literacy, what is financial literacy?

In the next section of the book, we will delve deeper into the important topics of financial literacy and land ownership and management. These two areas play a crucial role in shaping your family's financial health and stability, as well as facilitating long-term wealth-building and security.

First, we will explore financial literacy and its significance in helping individuals make informed financial decisions. Understanding key financial concepts, such as budgeting, saving, investing, and debt management, is essential for navigating the complex world of personal finance. We will discuss the importance of developing strong financial literacy skills and how they can empower you to achieve your financial goals, enhance your financial well-being, and secure a stable financial future for your family.

Next, we will shift our focus to land ownership and management, exploring the benefits and considerations associated with owning land. Land ownership can offer opportunities for wealth creation, income generation, and asset appreciation, but it also comes with responsibilities and potential challenges. We will discuss the various ways in which land ownership can impact your family's financial health and stability, as well as strategies for effectively managing and maximizing the financial potential of your land assets.

By combining insights into financial literacy and land ownership and management, this section of the book aims to provide you with valuable knowledge and practical guidance for strengthening your family's financial foundation, making sound financial decisions, and harnessing the potential of land ownership to build long-term financial security and prosperity. Stay tuned for in-depth discussions and expert insights on these important topics in the chapters ahead.

Financial literacy refers to the knowledge and skills required to make informed and effective financial decisions. It involves understanding fundamental financial concepts, such as budgeting, saving, investing, debt management, and retirement planning. Having a strong foundation in financial literacy can significantly impact your family's financial health and stability in several ways.

First and foremost, financial literacy enables individuals to make informed decisions about their finances, leading to better money management and planning for the future. By understanding concepts like budgeting and saving, families can develop effective financial habits that help them achieve their financial goals, such as building an emergency fund, paying off debt, or saving for retirement. Financial literacy also empowers individuals to make informed choices about financial products and services, such as insurance, investments, and loans, ensuring they select options that align with their needs and objectives.

Furthermore, financial literacy can help families navigate financial challenges and unexpected expenses more effectively. For example, households with higher levels of financial knowledge are better equipped to handle emergencies, manage debt responsibly, and withstand economic downturns. Additionally, financial literacy can improve communication about money within families, fostering open discussions about financial goals, priorities, and concerns.

Overall, financial literacy plays a crucial role in promoting the financial health and stability of a family. By equipping individuals with the knowledge and skills needed to make sound financial decisions, financial literacy can help families build a secure financial future, reduce financial stress, and achieve long-term financial well-being. Investing in financial education and improving financial literacy within your family can have lasting benefits and empower you to take control of your financial future.

Let's get financially fit! Here is a detailed list and summary of budgeting, saving, investing, debt management, and retirement planning, along with tips on how to do each of these effectively:

1. Budgeting:

- Budgeting is the process of creating a plan for your money, outlining your income and expenses.

- Start by tracking your income and expenses to understand your financial situation.

- Create a budget by allocating your income to different categories such as rent, groceries, utilities, savings, and entertainment.

- Regularly review and adjust your budget as needed to ensure you are on track to meet your financial goals.

2. Saving:

- Saving involves setting aside a portion of your income for future needs or emergencies.

- Establish an emergency fund with 3-6 months' worth of living expenses to cover unexpected costs.

- Save for short-term goals (e.g., vacation, new gadget) and long-term goals (e.g., buying a house, retirement).

- Automate your savings by setting up recurring transfers to a savings account.

3. Investing:

- Investing involves using your money to purchase assets that have the potential to grow in value over time.

- Understand your risk tolerance and investment goals before starting to invest.

- Diversify your investments across different asset classes (stocks, bonds, real estate) to reduce risk.

- Consider consulting with a financial advisor to help you make informed investment decisions.

4. Debt Management:

- Debt management involves effectively managing and paying off debt to improve your financial health.

- List out all your debts, including interest rates and minimum payments.

- Create a plan to pay off high-interest debts first while making minimum payments on others.

- Consider consolidating debts or negotiating with creditors to lower interest rates.

5. Retirement Planning:

- Retirement planning is the process of setting aside funds to support your lifestyle after retirement.

- Determine your retirement goals, such as desired retirement age and lifestyle.

- Contribute to retirement accounts like 401(k)s, IRAs, or Roth IRAs to build savings for retirement.

- Consider working with a financial planner to create a retirement plan tailored to your needs and goals.

Remember, each of these financial concepts is interconnected, and managing them effectively requires discipline, planning, and regular review of your financial situation. It's essential to stay informed about financial best practices and seek professional guidance when needed.

Now let us talk about annuities, bonds and stocks. Annuities are financial products offered by insurance companies that provide a guaranteed income stream for a specified period or for life, often used as a retirement income strategy. Stocks represent ownership in a company, offering the potential for capital appreciation and dividends but come with higher risks. Bonds are debt securities issued by governments or corporations, providing a fixed income stream through periodic interest payments and returning the principal amount at maturity. Balancing a portfolio with a mix of annuities, stocks, and bonds can help investors achieve diversification and manage risk based on their financial goals and risk tolerance levels.

Annuity

An annuity is a financial product that provides a series of payments at regular intervals, typically over a set period of time or for the rest of your life. There are different types of annuities, but the two main categories are immediate and deferred annuities. Immediate annuities start paying out right away, while deferred annuities accumulate funds over time before the payments begin.

One of the key benefits of annuities is their ability to offer a guaranteed income stream, providing financial security and peace of mind for you and your family. Annuities can be used as a tool for retirement planning, helping to supplement Social Security benefits, pension income, and other savings. They can also serve as a form of insurance against outliving your savings, as some annuities offer lifetime income options.

Additionally, annuities can provide tax advantages, such as tax-deferred growth on the earnings within the annuity until withdrawals are made. This can help with managing your tax liability, especially during retirement when income levels may be lower. Annuities can also offer flexibility in terms of payment options, beneficiaries, and customization to meet your specific financial goals and needs.

In summary, annuities can benefit your family's financial future by providing a reliable income stream, offering tax advantages, and helping to ensure financial security during retirement. They can serve as a valuable tool in a comprehensive financial plan, helping you to achieve your long-term financial goals and protect your loved ones' financial well-being.

Stocks

Stocks represent ownership in a company and are a type of investment that allows individuals to buy shares in a company, giving them a stake in its profits and losses. When you own stock in a company, you become a shareholder and may have the opportunity to receive dividends if the company distributes profits to its shareholders. The value of a stock fluctuates based on various factors, including company performance, market conditions, and investor sentiment. Investing in stocks can offer the potential for capital appreciation over time, as the value of the shares may increase, allowing you to sell them at a profit.

Stocks can benefit your family's financial future in several ways. First, investing in stocks has historically provided higher returns compared to other investment options, such as bonds or savings accounts, over the long term. This can help you grow your wealth and build a nest egg for your family's future financial needs, such as education expenses, home purchases, or retirement. Additionally, investing in a diversified portfolio of stocks can help you spread risk and mitigate potential losses, as the performance of individual stocks may vary.

Stocks also offer liquidity, meaning you can easily buy and sell shares on the stock market, providing flexibility to adjust your investment strategy based on your financial goals and market conditions.

In summary, investing in stocks can benefit your family's financial future by offering the potential for long-term growth, diversification, and liquidity. By incorporating stocks into your investment portfolio, you can work towards achieving financial goals, building wealth over time, and securing a stable financial foundation for your family's future needs. However, it's important to conduct thorough research, consider your risk tolerance, and consult with a financial advisor to develop a well-balanced investment strategy that aligns with your financial objectives and time horizon.

Bonds

Bonds are debt securities issued by governments, municipalities, or corporations to raise capital. When you purchase a bond, you are essentially lending money to the issuer in exchange for regular interest payments and the return of the principal amount at maturity. Bonds are considered a relatively safer investment compared to stocks because they provide a predictable income stream and are less volatile.

You can use bonds in your family's financial planning in various ways. For example, you can invest in government bonds or high-quality corporate bonds to preserve capital generate income for long-term financial goals such as education expenses, retirement savings, or buying a home. Bonds can also be used to diversify your investment portfolio, lower overall risk, and provide stability during market downturns. Additionally, bonds can serve as a conservative option for emergency funds or short-term savings goals, ensuring liquidity and capital preservation. Overall, incorporating bonds into your family's investment strategy can help protect and grow your wealth over time while providing peace of mind through stable income streams.

Now that we have discussed financial literacy, we will delve into land ownership and management.

Land ownership

Land ownership refers to the legal right to possess, use, and control a piece of land. Owning land can have significant implications for your family's financial health and stability, both in the short-term and long-term. Land ownership can provide various benefits and opportunities that can contribute to your family's financial well-being.

One of the primary advantages of land ownership is the potential for appreciation in value over time. Real estate, including land, has historically shown appreciation in value, making it a very valuable asset that can generate wealth for your family. Owning land can also offer opportunities for generating income, such as renting out the land for agricultural purposes, leasing it for commercial use, or developing it for residential or commercial properties. These income streams can provide a source of passive income for your family and contribute to financial stability.

Additionally, land ownership can serve as a form of security and stability for your family's financial future. Owning land provides a tangible asset that can be leveraged for collateral in obtaining loans or financing for other investments or expenses. Land ownership can also offer a sense of long-term stability and security, providing a place for your family to live, work, or retire, as well as potential inheritance for future generations.

However, land ownership also comes with responsibilities, such as property taxes, maintenance costs, and potential legal obligations. It is important to consider these factors when evaluating the financial implications of land ownership for your family. Proper planning and management of land ownership can help maximize the financial benefits while mitigating risks and ensuring long-term financial health and stability for your family. Land ownership and management entail a complex array of factors, responsibilities, and considerations. The process of land ownership typically begins with the legal acquisition of a property through purchase, inheritance, or other means. Once ownership is established, land management involves various tasks such as maintaining the property, complying with zoning regulations, paying property taxes, and adhering to environmental regulations. Effective land management also includes optimizing land use for agricultural, residential, commercial, or conservation purposes. Landowners may need to consider factors such as soil quality, water resources, topography, and biodiversity when making decisions about land management practices. Additionally, land management often involves addressing issues such as erosion control, pest management, habitat conservation, and sustainable resource use. Overall, successful land ownership and management requires a combination of legal knowledge, thoughtful planning, environmental stewardship, and sound decision-making to ensure the long-term health and productivity of the land. Who doesn't want to own their own, right? It is a part of your family legacy and healthy lifestyle.

Part 5: Mom and Dad

Chapter Nine: Collectively Embracing a Healthy Lifestyle

Chapter Nine: Collectively Embracing a Healthy Lifestyle

Cultivating a Healthy Relationship and Lifestyle for the Benefit of the Family.

In this pivotal chapter, we delve into the integral role of husband and wife in fostering a nurturing and supportive relationship built on mutual respect, communication, and shared values. By prioritizing their well-being and collectively embracing a healthy lifestyle, they not only enrich their own lives but also create a harmonious environment that benefits the entire family unit.

Building a Strong Foundation of Communication and Trust

Communication forms the cornerstone of a healthy relationship between husband and wife. By fostering open and honest communication, they create a safe space for sharing thoughts, feelings, and concerns. Regular conversations that involve active listening and empathy help strengthen their bond and build trust within the relationship. Mutual respect for each other's perspectives and a willingness to compromise ensure that conflicts are addressed constructively, fostering a sense of unity, and understanding. You're not going to always agree but there's a healthy way to verbally fight.

Prioritizing Emotional Well-Being and Support

Emotional support is essential in maintaining a healthy relationship and lifestyle. Husband and wife should be attuned to each other's emotional needs, offering comfort, encouragement, and reassurance during challenging times. By practicing empathy and being emotionally present for one another, they cultivate a sense of security and belonging within the relationship. Seeking professional help or counseling when needed further strengthens their emotional connection and equips them with the tools to navigate life's ups and downs together.

Embracing a Healthy Lifestyle Together

A healthy lifestyle is not just about individual choices but a shared commitment that husband and wife can embark on together. By prioritizing physical health through regular exercise, balanced nutrition, and adequate rest, they set a positive example for their family and create a foundation for long-term well-being. Engaging in activities such as outdoor walks, cooking nutritious meals together, or practicing mindfulness exercises fosters a sense of partnership and shared goals in promoting a healthy lifestyle.

Nurturing Personal Growth and Connection

Individual growth and self-care are pivotal in maintaining a healthy relationship. Husband and wife should prioritize their own personal development, hobbies, and interests, while also making time for shared experiences that deepen their connection. Engaging in activities that promote self-discovery, such as journaling, meditation, or pursuing new skills, allows each partner to flourish personally and bring a renewed sense of fulfillment and energy to their relationship.

Creating a Supportive Family Environment

A strong and healthy relationship between husband and wife sets the foundation for a supportive family environment. By modeling effective communication, respect, and care for one another, they demonstrate to their children the importance of love and mutual understanding. Shared family activities, traditions, and values further solidify the bond between husband and wife, creating a nurturing atmosphere where each family member feels valued, heard, and loved.

In cultivating a healthy relationship and lifestyle between husband and wife is not only beneficial for their own well-being but also contributes to the overall harmony and happiness of the family. By prioritizing communication, trust, emotional support, and shared experiences, they lay the groundwork for a resilient partnership that stands the test of time and serves as a source of strength and inspiration for generations to come.

Healthy ways for couples to engage in verbal fights:

Healthy communication is essential in any relationship, including during disagreements or conflicts. When couples engage in verbal disagreements, it's important to approach the situation with respect, empathy, and a willingness to work towards resolution. Here are some healthy ways for couples to engage in verbal fights:

1. Choose the Right Time and Place:

Pick a suitable time and place to have a constructive conversation. Avoid discussing sensitive topics when either partner is tired, stressed, or distracted. Find a quiet setting where both individuals can focus on the discussion without interruptions.

2. Use "I" Statements:

Frame your thoughts and feelings using "I" statements to express your perspective without blaming or accusing your partner. For example, say "I feel hurt when..." instead of "You always make me feel..." This helps prevent defensiveness and allows for better understanding.

3. Practice Active Listening:

Listen attentively to your partner's concerns without interrupting or formulating your response. Show empathy by reflecting on what your partner is saying to ensure that you understand their feelings and perspective.

4. Take Breaks When Needed:

If emotions escalate or tensions run high during the discussion, it's okay to take a break. Agree on a time to revisit the conversation after both individuals have had a chance to calm down and collect their thoughts.

5. Focus on the Issue, Not the Person:

Keep the discussion centered on the specific issue at hand rather than resorting to personal attacks or criticisms. Recognize that disagreements are natural, and the goal is to find a solution together, not to assign blame.

6. Practice Validation and Empathy:

Validate your partner's feelings by acknowledging their perspective, even if you may not agree with it. Express empathy and understanding towards their emotions, demonstrating that you value their feelings and experiences.

7. Seek Compromise and Solutions:

Approach the disagreement with a mindset of finding common ground and seeking solutions that benefit both partners. Be open to compromise and brainstorming ideas that address the needs and concerns of one another.

8. Use "We" Language:

Shift the conversation towards shared goals and mutual understanding by using "we" language. Focus on working together as a team to resolve conflicts and strengthen the relationship.

9. Express Appreciation and Affection:

After resolving the disagreement, take the time to express appreciation for your partner's willingness to communicate openly and work towards resolution. Show affection and reaffirm your commitment to the relationship.

10. Seek Professional Help if Needed:

If verbal fights become frequent or escalate into unhealthy patterns, consider seeking the support of a couple's therapist or counselor. Professional guidance can provide valuable tools and strategies for improving communication and conflict resolution within the relationship.

By incorporating these healthy practices into verbal fights, couples can navigate disagreements with respect, understanding, and a shared commitment to strengthening their relationship. Open communication, active listening, empathy, and a focus on finding solutions can help couples resolve conflicts constructively and foster a deeper connection with each other.

Couples: Maintaining a good sexual relationship

Maintaining a good sexual relationship can have numerous positive effects on a marriage and family dynamics. Healthy and satisfying sexual intimacy fosters emotional closeness, strengthens the bond between partners, and increases feelings of love and connection. This, in turn, can lead to improved communication, trust, and overall relationship satisfaction. Couples who are regularly intimate often experience lower levels of stress and anxiety, leading to a more harmonious and supportive environment at home. A robust sexual relationship can also enhance physical and mental well-being, as intimacy releases endorphins and promotes relaxation. Additionally, a strong connection between partners can serve as a positive role model for children, demonstrating the importance of mutual respect, communication, and affection in a loving relationship. Overall, a good sexual relationship can contribute to a happy and stable marriage, creating a strong foundation for a healthy and thriving family unit.

How to ensure a healthy sexual Relationship

Couples can ensure a healthy sexual relationship by prioritizing communication, mutual respect, and emotional intimacy. Open and honest communication about desires, boundaries, and concerns is essential for both partners to feel heard and understood. Building trust and respect within the relationship creates a safe space for exploring each other's needs and preferences. Cultivating emotional intimacy through quality time together, shared activities, and deep conversations can strengthen the bond between partners and enhance their sexual connection. To improve their sexual relationship, couples can try the following ways:

1. Prioritize physical touch and affection outside the bedroom to maintain connection and intimacy.

2. Explore new activities or experiences together to keep the spark alive and enhance excitement.

3. Experiment with different techniques, positions, or fantasies to spice up the sexual routine.

4. Seek professional help or attend therapy sessions if facing difficulties or challenges in the bedroom.

5. Practice mindfulness and focus on being present during intimate moments to deepen connection and pleasure.

6. Schedule regular date nights or romantic getaways to rekindle romance and passion in the relationship.

7. Invest in self-care and prioritize individual well-being to feel more confident and satisfied in the relationship.

By implementing these strategies and investing time and effort into their sexual relationship, couples can strengthen their bond, deepen intimacy, and enjoy a fulfilling and healthy connection.

Couples bonding and romance

Building a strong bond and keeping the romance alive in a relationship are essential components for a lasting and fulfilling partnership. A strong bond between partners fosters trust, communication, and emotional intimacy, creating a solid foundation for a successful relationship. Additionally, maintaining romance keeps the spark alive, reigniting and excitement in the. Overall, investing in couples bonding and nurturing romance helps partners deepen their connection, strengthen their commitment to each other, and create a relationship with love, joy, and fulfillment.

Couples! Building a strong and healthy relationship takes effort from both partners. Here are some detailed ways for a couple to ensure their bonding and the relationship is strong:

1. Communication: Effective communication is key in any relationship. Take the time to listen to each other, express your feelings openly, and work together to resolve conflicts peacefully.

2. Quality time together: Make time for each other regularly, whether it's going on dates, taking walks, cooking together, or simply relaxing at home. Spending quality time together strengthens the emotional bond between partners.

3. Shared interests and activities: Find activities or hobbies that you both enjoy and engage in them together. This can create shared experiences and memories that help deepen your connection.

4. Show appreciation and gratitude: Express your appreciation for each other regularly. Acknowledge and thank your partner for the things they do and show gratitude for their presence in your life.

5. Trust and honesty: Build a foundation of trust by being open and honest with each other. Trust is essential for a strong relationship, so avoid keeping secrets and be trustworthy in your actions.

6. Respect: Treat each other with respect always, even during disagreements. Respect each other's opinions, boundaries, and feelings, and avoid belittling or disrespecting your partner.

7. Support each other: Be there for your partner during both the good times and the challenging times. Offer emotional support, encouragement, and understanding when needed.

8. Work as a team: Approach challenges and decisions as a team, with both partners contributing equally. Collaborate on problem-solving and goal setting to strengthen your partnership.

9. Physical intimacy: Physical affection and intimacy are important aspects of a romantic relationship. Find ways to connect physically, whether through hugs, kisses, cuddling, or sexual intimacy.

10. Practice forgiveness: Forgiveness is crucial in maintaining a healthy relationship. Learn to forgive each other's mistakes, let go of grudges, and move forward together with a renewed focus on growth and improvement.

In trying these in your relationship, you can strengthen the bond between you and your partner and ensure that your relationship remains strong and satisfying.

Keeping the romance alive

Keeping the romance alive in a relationship requires ongoing effort and creativity. Here are some detailed ways for a couple to ensure they maintain a sense of romance:

1. Date nights: Regularly schedule date nights to spend quality time together without distractions. This could involve going out to a nice restaurant, watching a movie, or trying a new activity together.

2. Surprise gestures: Keep the element of surprise alive by occasionally surprising your partner with thoughtful gestures, such as love notes, small gifts, or unexpected acts of kindness.

3. Physical affection: Make sure to maintain physical affection in your relationship, whether through hugs, kisses, holding hands, or cuddling. Physical touch helps to foster a sense of intimacy and closeness.

4. Keep the spark alive: Continuously work on keeping the spark alive by flirting with your partner, complimenting them, and finding ways to show your attraction and desire for them.

5. Spontaneity: Embrace spontaneity by breaking out of routines and trying new things together. This could involve planning spontaneous weekend getaways, trying a new hobby, or exploring your city in a new way.

6. Communicate openly about your needs: Have open and honest conversations about your needs and desires in the relationship. Understanding each other's love languages and preferences can help you keep the romance alive in a way that resonates with both partners.

7. Keep romance alive in everyday moments: Find ways to infuse romance into your everyday interactions, such as by leaving sweet messages, cooking a special meal together, or creating a cozy atmosphere at home.

8. Shared experiences: Try some new things together, whether it's traveling to a new destination, attending a concert, or taking a cooking , dancing or art class. Shared experiences help to strengthen the bond between partners.

9. Express appreciation: Show your partner how much you appreciate them by expressing gratitude for the things they do, acknowledging their efforts, and recognizing their positive qualities.

10. Invest in self-care: Take care of yourself individually to maintain a sense of confidence and well-being in the relationship. When both partners prioritize self-care, it contributes to a healthier and more fulfilling relationship overall.

By trying these out, you can solidify that the romance remains alive and thriving, keeping the love between you and your partner strong and vibrant. Couples bonding and keeping the romance alive are vital aspects of a successful and fulfilling relationship. Building a strong bond through communication, shared experiences, and trust fosters emotional intimacy and connection between mates. Additionally, maintaining romance through gestures, quality time, and physical affection helps keep the spark alive and ignites passion in the relationship. Always prioritizing these elements, couples can enhance their relationship, strengthen their connection, and create a lasting partnership filled with love and happiness.

My husband one day years ago told me that making love is an all-day process. It still rings true to this day. From good morning kisses to unexpected touches, compliments to cooked and shared meals. We can't forget about the naughty text messages, the sexy picture messages and flirting throughout the day, it's all making love to the mind and body.

"Making love is an all-day process."- E. Williams

This chapter underscores the importance of husband and wife working together to nurture a healthy relationship and lifestyle for the benefit of the family. By prioritizing communication, support, shared goals, and personal growth, they create a foundation of love and unity that enriches both their lives and the well-being of their family. Children simulate their parents, striving to be like them in every way as a child. Take that into consideration as you go about your days of actions and deeds.

If dad and mom's relationship is toxic it breeds an unhealthy family and creates a venomous generational cycle. Which is a very hard thing to endure and change. I am someone who struggled with trying to break one of many of my own family's generational curses or cycles. I have referred to it by both terms at different points of the challenges. Understand that there is no set time frame for overcoming and conquering those cycles, there's no perfect way to achieve it either. Looking for perfection is no help and there is no quick fix. I learned the hard way that it does take time and not in your desired time frame. Be strong! It is best to have your relationship together and consistently grow before starting a family. It helps you in the long run to avoid having to learn those lessons later when you're having to deal with whatever life is throwing at you at that time.

Congratulations if you are considering starting your family. Keep reading in the next section I'll talk about just that.

The Joys of Starting a Family

Starting a family is a transformative and soul-enriching experience that brings immense joy, love, and happiness into the lives of couples. From the moment you decide to expand your family to the arrival of your precious little one and the journey of parenthood that follows, the joys of starting a family are truly unparalleled. In this chapter, we will explore the profound moments of joy and happiness that come with embarking on the beautiful adventure of creating a family.

1. Shared Excitement and Anticipation:

The decision to start a family is often met with shared excitement and anticipation between partners. The joy of imagining your future as parents, envisioning the bond you will share with your child, and planning for the arrival of a new family member can create a sense of unity, purpose, and love that strengthens your relationship and deepens your connection with each other.

2. Wonder and Amazement of Pregnancy:

Pregnancy is a miraculous journey filled with wonder and amazement as you witness the growth and development of your unborn child. Feeling the first kicks, hearing the heartbeat for the first time, seeing ultrasound images of your baby's tiny features — these moments of joy and anticipation create a profound sense of love and connection between you and your growing family.

3. Bonding with Your Baby:

The moment your child is born and placed in your arms is a pure and unparalleled experience of joy and happiness. The bond that forms between you and your baby in those precious first moments is indescribable, as you gaze into their eyes, hold them close, and feel an overwhelming sense of love and protection. The simple joys of feeding, soothing, and cuddling your baby create a deep sense of fulfillment and purpose that enriches your life in ways you never imagined.

4. Milestones and Memories:

Watching your child grow and reach new milestones is a source of boundless joy and pride for parents. From their first smile to their first words, first steps, and beyond, every moment of discovery and achievement fills your heart with happiness and gratitude. Capturing these precious moments through photos, videos, and shared experiences creates lasting memories that you will cherish for a lifetime.

5. Unconditional Love and Support:

The joy of starting a family is rooted in the unconditional love, support, and connection that parents share with their children. Through the challenges, triumphs, laughter, and tears that come with parenthood, the deep love and bond that you cultivate with your child create a sense of fulfillment and joy that sustains you through every stage of the journey.

To come to the point, the joy and happiness that come with starting a family are immeasurable and enduring. From the shared excitement of planning for a new chapter in your lives to the profound moments of love, connection, and growth that unfold as you welcome a child into your family, the joys of parenthood are a gift that unfolds with each passing day. Embrace the journey with gratitude, openness, and a heart full of love, and savor every moment of joy and happiness that comes with building a family together. So really take the time to think about all the other things that come with the joy in the journey.

The Journey of Child Planning

As a couple embarks on the passage of building a family, the decision to have children is a significant milestone that requires thoughtful consideration, planning, and preparation. Bringing a child into the world is a deeply fulfilling experience that can bring immense joy and fulfillment to a couple's life. However, it is important for couples to enter this decision with open communication, shared goals, and a solid foundation to nurture a growing family.

Before diving into the process of child planning, couples should take the time to reflect on their personal readiness and readiness as a couple to take on the responsibilities of parenthood. Considerations such as emotional maturity, financial stability, career goals, and relationship dynamics all play a crucial role in determining if the timing is right to start a family.

One of the first steps in child planning is to have open and honest conversations about your desires, fears, and expectations regarding parenthood. Discuss your individual values, beliefs, and parenting styles to ensure that you are on the same page when it comes to raising a child. It is important to establish mutual goals and priorities for your family to create a shared vision for the future.

Financial planning is another key aspect of child planning that cannot be overlooked. Children come with a range of financial responsibilities, including healthcare expenses, education costs, childcare, and everyday living expenses. Take the time to assess your current financial situation and create a budget that accounts for the additional expenses that come with raising a child. Consider creating a savings plan or setting aside a fund specifically for your future child's needs.

Beyond the practical considerations, couples should also prepare themselves emotionally and mentally for the challenges and joys of parenthood. Understand that having a child will bring changes to your lifestyle, routines, and priorities. It is important to cultivate patience, flexibility, and resilience to navigate the ups and downs that come with raising a child.

Once you have made the decision to start a family, consider seeking guidance from healthcare professionals to ensure a smooth and healthy pregnancy. Visit your doctor for preconception counseling, prenatal care, and genetic testing to address any potential risks or concerns before conception. Take steps to optimize your health by adopting a healthy lifestyle, including regular exercise, balanced nutrition, and adequate rest.

Now, the journey of child planning is a deeply personal and enriching experience that requires careful consideration, preparation, and teamwork from both partners. By prioritizing open communication, shared goals, financial planning, emotional readiness, and healthcare guidance, couples can embark on the path to parenthood with confidence and excitement for the future. Remember that parenthood is a journey filled with love, challenges, and endless rewards that will forever change your lives in the most beautiful ways. Okay so now let's breakdown the financial aspect of having a baby. Yes, it is a necessary thought, like the old heads said it. "No romance without finance" or "No money no honey". I know it might not sound right but if you think about it, it's kind of true. I said that to say this, it takes money to have and raise a child, and it's not cheap. In the next section I will break it down a bit for you.

Financial Considerations for Starting a Family

As a couple prepares to start a family, it is crucial to understand and plan for the various expenses that come with raising children. From pregnancy and childbirth costs to ongoing childcare, education, and healthcare expenses, the financial responsibilities of parenthood can have a significant impact on a couple's budget and financial security. In this chapter, we will explore the key expenses that couples should consider when starting a family and offer tips on how to manage them effectively.

1. Pregnancy and Childbirth Costs:

Pregnancy and childbirth can be accompanied by a range of expenses, including prenatal care, delivery fees, hospital charges, and postnatal care for both the mother and the newborn. It is essential to factor in these expenses and determine how they will be covered by your health insurance or personal savings. Consider creating a budget specifically for pregnancy-related costs to ensure that you are financially prepared for this significant life event.

2. Childcare Expenses:

One of the most significant ongoing expenses of raising a family is childcare. Whether you choose to enroll your child in a daycare center, hire a nanny, or have a family member provide care, childcare costs can quickly add up. Research different childcare options in your area, compare costs, and create a budget that includes these expenses. You may also be eligible for tax credits or employer-sponsored childcare benefits to help offset some of these costs.

3. Education Costs:

Planning for your child's education is another important financial consideration for starting a family. Costs associated with preschool, private school tuition, extracurricular activities, and higher education can put a strain on your finances if not planned for in advance. Consider opening a college savings account, such as a 529 plan, to start saving for your child's future education expenses early on. Explore scholarship opportunities, financial aid options, and educational tax benefits to help lessen the burden of education costs.

4. Healthcare Expenses:

Healthcare expenses for your child, including routine doctor visits, vaccinations, dental care, and unexpected medical emergencies, are an essential part of your family's budget. Make sure you have adequate health insurance coverage that includes your child's medical needs and understand your out-of-pocket costs for healthcare services. Consider setting aside a healthcare fund or emergency savings account to cover unexpected medical expenses that may arise.

5. Everyday Living Expenses:

Beyond the specific costs mentioned above, starting a family also entails everyday living expenses such as food, clothing, housing, utilities, transportation, and entertainment. Factor in these expenses when creating your family budget and look for ways to save money through smart shopping, meal planning, energy-efficient practices, and budget-friendly activities.

In conclusion, starting a family involves a range of financial considerations that require careful planning, budgeting, and prioritization. By understanding the key expenses associated with raising children and taking proactive steps to manage your finances effectively, you can create a solid financial foundation for your growing family. Remember to communicate openly with your partner, seek financial guidance when needed, and make informed decisions that align with your family's values and goals. With proper financial planning and a commitment to financial responsibility, you can navigate the expenses of starting a family with confidence and security.

In summing up, starting your family is a deeply rewarding and life-changing experience that brings a blend of emotions, challenges, and joys. It begins with a couple's decision to expand their family, requiring thoughtful consideration of readiness, communication, and financial planning. The journey of child planning involves discussing values, setting shared goals, and preparing emotionally and mentally for the responsibilities of parenthood.

Financial considerations play a significant role in starting a family, as couples must budget for pregnancy and childbirth costs, ongoing childcare expenses, education costs, healthcare expenses, and everyday living expenses. By creating a financial plan, setting priorities, and seeking guidance when needed, couples can navigate the expenses of raising a family with confidence and security.

Despite the inevitable challenges that come with starting a family, the sheer joy and happiness that accompany parenthood are unmatched. From the shared excitement and anticipation of starting a family to the wonder and amazement of pregnancy, bonding with your baby, celebrating milestones and creating lasting memories, the joys of parenthood are profound and heartwarming. Through the unconditional love, support, and connection that parents share with their children, the journey of starting a family is filled with moments of love, growth, and fulfillment that shape the lives of couples in the most beautiful ways.

Part 6: Building Blocks of Wellness

Chapter Ten: Empowering Kids: Strategies for Life

Chapter Ten: Empowering Kids: Strategies for Life

Empowering kids for a healthy future is crucial to help them lead fulfilling lives and reduce the risk of developing chronic health problems later in life. By instilling healthy habits and promoting physical activity, children are better equipped with the tools to make positive lifestyle choices. Strategies for lifelong wellness, such as promoting a balanced diet, encouraging regular exercise, and prioritizing mental health, play a significant role in shaping a child's overall well-being. These strategies not only have immediate benefits for physical health but also contribute to strong cognitive development and emotional resilience. By emphasizing the importance of health and wellness from a young age, we are laying the foundation for children to lead happier, healthier lives long into adulthood.

Promoting a balanced diet

A child's physical health can be supported through a balanced diet rich in fruits, vegetables, whole grains, and lean proteins. A child's balanced diet should include a variety of nutrient-rich foods to support their growth and development. Here is a descriptive list of examples of foods that can be part of a child's balanced diet:

1. Fruits: Include a variety of fresh fruits such as apples, bananas, berries, oranges, and melons to provide essential vitamins, minerals, and fiber.

2. Vegetables: Offer a colorful array of vegetables like spinach, carrots, broccoli, bell peppers, and sweet potatoes to ensure a good intake of vitamins, minerals, and antioxidants.

3. Whole grains: Incorporate whole grain foods like whole wheat bread, brown rice, oats, and whole grain pasta for fiber, energy, and essential nutrients.

4. Protein: Include lean sources of protein such as chicken, turkey, fish, eggs, tofu, beans, and lentils for muscle development and overall growth.

5. Dairy: Provide calcium-rich dairy products like milk, yogurt, and cheese to support bone health and growth.

6. Healthy fats: Include sources of healthy fats such as avocado, nuts, seeds, and olive oil for brain development and overall health.

7. Water: Encourage drinking plenty of water throughout the day to stay hydrated and support overall health.

Making these foods available for a child's diet, you can ensure they are receiving a well-rounded and nutritionally balanced meal plan. Bare in mind kids like choices so, plenty healthy food options make eating fun, your job easier and your kids healthier.

Encouraging regular exercise

It is crucial for children to engage in healthy activities for their overall well-being and development. Physical activities such as running, jumping, playing sports, and participating in outdoor games are essential for promoting good physical health, building strong muscles and bones, and improving cardiovascular fitness. Additionally, participating in healthy activities can help children maintain a healthy weight, reduce the risk of developing chronic conditions like obesity and diabetes, and improve their overall physical stamina and endurance. Beyond the physical benefits, engaging in healthy activities also has positive effects on children's mental health, as it can reduce stress, improve mood, boost self-esteem, enhance cognitive function, and foster social skills through interaction with peers. Encouraging children to lead an active lifestyle from a young age sets the foundation for lifelong habits of health and wellness.

Healthy activities for children

1. Outdoor sports: Engage in activities such as soccer, basketball, volleyball, or tennis that promote physical fitness, coordination, and teamwork.

2. Hiking: Explore nature trails, parks, or local forests together as a family, allowing children to appreciate the outdoors and enjoy the benefits of fresh air and physical activity.

3. Biking: Take family bike rides around the neighborhood or on designated biking trails to improve cardiovascular health and strengthen leg muscles.

4. Swimming: Visit a local pool, beach, or water park for a fun and refreshing activity that provides a full-body workout and helps build endurance and coordination.

5. Gardening: Involve children in planting and tending to a family garden, teaching them about healthy eating, responsibility, and the importance of connecting with nature.

6. Dance party: Have a dance-off in the living room to get everyone moving and grooving while improving coordination, flexibility, and mood.

7. Yoga: Practice yoga poses together as a family to promote mindfulness, flexibility, balance, and relaxation.

8. Family fitness challenges: Create friendly competitions or challenges that encourage physical activity, such as a timed obstacle course, jumping jacks contest, or push-up challenge.

9. Picnics: Pack healthy snacks and meals for a picnic in the park or backyard, combining outdoor relaxation with physical activities like frisbee, tag, or kite flying.

10. Family workout sessions: Dedicate time for family exercise routines like aerobics, strength training, or stretching, promoting fitness, bonding, and overall health and well-being.

Engaging in healthy activities as a child and as a family has far-reaching benefits for overall well-being. Physical activities such as exercise, sports, outdoor play, and recreational pursuits have a positive impact on physical health by promoting strength, endurance, flexibility, and cardiovascular fitness. These activities also help children and families maintain a healthy weight, reduce the risk of chronic diseases, and improve overall physical well-being.

In addition to the physical benefits, participating in healthy activities can boost mental health by reducing stress, anxiety, and depression, improving mood, enhancing cognitive function, and promoting better sleep patterns. Healthy activities also provide opportunities for families to bond, communicate, and create lasting memories together, strengthening relationships and fostering a sense of unity and connection. Furthermore, engaging in healthy activities as a family can instill important values such as teamwork, perseverance, discipline, and goal setting, which are beneficial for personal growth and character development. Overall, incorporating healthy activities into the daily routine of children and families can lead to improved physical health, mental well-being, emotional resilience, social connections, and overall quality of life.

Prioritizing mental health

Prioritizing children's mental health is essential for their overall well-being and development. As parents and or caregivers, there are several ways we can help support children's mental health. Creating a safe and nurturing environment where children feel heard, understood, and valued is crucial. Encouraging open communication and actively listening to their thoughts and feelings can help them express themselves and manage stress or anxiety effectively. Providing opportunities for physical activity, creative expression, and relaxation can also contribute to a positive mental state. It is important to model healthy coping skills and self-care practices to show children how to manage emotions and build resilience. Additionally, seeking professional help when needed and destigmatizing mental health challenges can ensure that children receive the support they need to thrive emotionally and mentally. By prioritizing children's mental health and offering them the tools and resources to navigate their emotions, we can help them develop into emotionally intelligent and resilient individuals.

The mental and emotional stages of childhood

During childhood, mental and emotional development progresses through various stages, each with its own characteristics and milestones. Here is a detailed summary and list of the mental and emotional stages of childhood:

1. Infancy (0-2 years): Infants develop trust and bond with their caregivers. They begin to form basic attachments and learn to regulate their emotions through interactions with their primary caregivers.

2. Early Childhood (2-6 years): Children in this stage develop a sense of autonomy and independence. They are curious and eager to explore the world around them. They begin to develop social skills and learn to identify and express their emotions.

3. Middle Childhood (6-12 years): During this stage, children start to develop a sense of industry and competence.

They become more aware of social norms and expectations and form relationships outside the family. Children also start to understand the perspectives of others and improve their communication skills.

4. Adolescence (12-18 years): Adolescents go through significant changes in identity and social relationships. They start to question authority, develop more complex emotions, and seek independence. Adolescence is a period of self-discovery, where teenagers form their beliefs, values, and goals for the future.

Each stage of childhood has unique challenges and opportunities for mental and emotional growth. Parents, caregivers, and educators play a vital role in supporting children through these stages by providing guidance, encouragement, and a safe space for exploration and expression.

Regular check-ups

Regular check-ups with healthcare providers, including vaccinations, can help prevent illness and ensure proper growth and development. Regular check-ups for kids are essential for monitoring their growth, development, and overall health. These appointments allow healthcare providers to track important milestones, ensure that children are growing and developing appropriately, and detect any potential health issues early on. Regular check-ups also provide an opportunity for vaccinations to be administered, helping to protect children from serious illnesses. These appointments offer a chance for parents to ask questions, address any concerns, and receive guidance on important topics such as nutrition, safety, and behavior. By scheduling regular check-ups for their children, parents can take proactive steps towards ensuring their kids' well-being and setting them up for a healthy future.

Some common children's diseases to look out for in your child's childhood:

1. Chickenpox: Chickenpox is a highly contagious viral infection that causes an itchy rash with small, red spots. It usually starts on the back, chest, and face, and then spreads to the rest of the body. Children may also have a fever and feel unwell.

2. Measles: Measles is a viral infection that causes a red, blotchy rash all over the body, along with fever, cough, runny nose, and red, watery eyes. Measles can be serious and lead to complications, so vaccination is important.

3. Mumps: Mumps are a viral infection that causes swelling of the salivary glands, leading to puffy cheeks and a swollen jaw. Children with mumps may also have fever, headache, and muscle aches.

4. Rubella (German Measles): Rubella is a viral infection that causes a mild rash, low fever, and swollen lymph nodes. Pregnant women who contract rubella are at risk of passing the infection to their unborn baby, which can lead to serious birth defects.

5. Whooping Cough (Pertussis): Whooping cough is a highly contagious bacterial infection that causes severe coughing fits, often accompanied by a "whooping" sound when trying to breathe in. It can be especially serious in young children and infants.

6. Scarlet Fever: Scarlet fever is a bacterial infection that can cause a red rash with a sandpaper-like texture, along with high fever, sore throat, and swollen glands. It is caused by the same bacteria that causes strep throat.

7. Hand, Foot, and Mouth Disease: Hand, foot, and mouth disease is a viral infection that causes a rash on the hands, feet, and in the mouth. It is common in young children and can cause fever, sore throat, and general discomfort.

8. Roseola: Roseola is a viral infection that causes high fever followed by a pink rash on the trunk and spreading to the arms, legs, and neck. Children with roseola may also have a runny nose and mild cough.

9. Fifth Disease (Erythema Infectiosum): Fifth disease is a viral infection that causes a "slapped cheek" rash on the face, as well as a lacy rash on the arms and legs. It is typically a mild illness but can be more serious for pregnant women.

10. Croup: Croup is a viral infection that causes swelling in the voice box and windpipe, leading to a barking cough and noisy breathing. It most commonly affects young children and can be frightening but is usually not serious.

It is important to monitor your child for any signs or symptoms of these diseases and consult with a healthcare provider if you suspect they may be ill. Vaccinations and good hygiene practices can help prevent many of these childhood diseases.

Here is a list of common children's diseases and their associated treatments:

1. Chickenpox:

- Treatment: Chickenpox is a viral illness that typically resolves on its own within 1-2 weeks. Treatment focuses on relieving symptoms, such as fever and itching. Over-the-counter medications like acetaminophen can help reduce fever and discomfort. Calamine lotion or oatmeal baths can help soothe itchy skin.

2. Measles:

- Treatment: There is no specific treatment for measles, so supportive care is typically recommended. Rest, hydration, and managing fever with acetaminophen are important.

Complications may require additional treatment, such as antibiotics for secondary bacterial infections.

3. Mumps:

- Treatment: Like measles, mumps do not have a specific treatment. Treatment focuses on managing symptoms, such as pain and fever. Rest, hydration, and over-the-counter pain relievers can help ease discomfort. In severe cases, hospitalization may be necessary.

4. Rubella (German Measles):

- Treatment: Rubella is typically a mild illness that resolves on its own. Rest and supportive care are important. Pregnant women should avoid contact with individuals who have rubella to prevent transmission to the fetus.

5. Whooping Cough (Pertussis):

- Treatment: Treatment for whooping cough usually involves a course of antibiotics to help reduce the severity and duration of the illness. Supportive care, such as rest, hydration, and monitoring for respiratory distress, is also important.

6. Scarlet Fever:

- Treatment: Scarlet fever is treated with antibiotics to eliminate the streptococcal bacteria causing the infection. The course of antibiotics must be completed as prescribed to prevent complications like rheumatic fever or kidney damage.

7. Hand, Foot, and Mouth Disease:

- Treatment: Hand, foot, and mouth disease is a viral illness that typically resolves on its own within a week. Treatment focuses on managing symptoms, such as fever and mouth ulcers. Over-the-counter pain relievers can help ease discomfort.

8. Roseola:

- Treatment: Roseola is a viral illness that is usually mild and self-limiting. Treatment focuses on managing fever and providing comfort measures, such as rest and hydration. Over-the-counter medications may be used to reduce fever if needed.

9. Fifth Disease (Erythema Infectiosum):

- Treatment: Fifth disease is typically a mild illness that does not require specific treatment. Supportive care, such as rest and hydration, can help manage symptoms. Pregnant women should consult with their healthcare provider if exposed to the virus.

10. Croup:

- Treatment: Mild cases of croup can be managed at home with humidified air, hydration, and comforting your child. Severe cases may require medical intervention, such as corticosteroids or nebulized medications, to reduce airway inflammation and improve breathing.

Always consult with a healthcare provider for an accurate diagnosis and appropriate treatment plan for your child's specific condition.

Vaccine-preventable diseases along with brief descriptions of each:

1. Measles: A highly contagious viral infection that causes rash, fever, cough, runny nose, and red, watery eyes. Complications can include pneumonia, encephalitis, and in severe cases, death.

2. Polio: A viral infection that can cause permanent paralysis, muscle weakness, and in severe cases, death. It spreads through contaminated food and water.

3. Mumps: A viral infection that results in swelling of the salivary glands, fever, headache, muscle aches, and fatigue. Complications can include deafness, meningitis, and infertility in males.

4. Rubella (German measles): A viral infection that causes a mild rash, fever, and swollen lymph nodes. If a pregnant woman gets infected, it can lead to serious birth defects in the fetus.

5. Varicella (Chickenpox): A highly contagious viral infection that causes itchy, blister-like rash, fever, and fatigue. Complications can include bacterial infections, pneumonia, and enalitis.

6. Hepatitis B: A viral infection that affects the liver and can lead to chronic liver disease, liver failure, and liver cancer. It is spread through contact with infected blood or bodily fluids.

7. Influenza (Flu): A respiratory illness caused by influenza viruses that can result in fever, cough, sore throat, muscle aches, and fatigue. In severe cases, it can lead to pneumonia and death.

8. Pertussis (Whooping Cough): A bacterial respiratory infection that causes severe coughing fits, vomiting, and difficulty breathing. It can be especially dangerous for infants.

9. Tetanus: A bacterial infection that causes muscle stiffness and spasms, often leading to difficulty swallowing and breathing. It enters the body through cuts or wounds contaminated with soil or manure.

10. Haemophilus influenzae type b (Hib): A bacterial infection that can cause serious diseases such as meningitis, pneumonia, and sepsis in young children. It spreads through respiratory droplets.

Vaccines have been developed to these diseases by stimulating the body's immune response to produce antibodies that can fight off the infection. Keeping up to date with recommended vaccinations can help protect individuals and communities from these potentially serious and sometimes deadly diseases.

Pediatric doctors use regular check-ups as a crucial form of preventative care to monitor the health and well-being of children. By scheduling routine appointments, pediatricians can track a child's growth and development over time, detecting any potential issues early on. Through thorough physical examinations, screenings, and discussions with parents, pediatric doctors can assess a child's overall health and identify any risk factors or concerns that may require further evaluation or intervention. Regular check-ups also provide an opportunity for vaccines to be administered, protecting children from serious diseases. Additionally, these visits allow pediatricians to offer guidance on nutrition, safety, and behavior, empowering parents with the information they need to promote their child's optimal health and development. Emphasizing the importance of regular check-ups as preventative care helps to ensure that children stay healthy and thrive as they grow.

Inspiring spiritual growth

Children's spiritual growth plays a significant role in their overall development and well-being, encompassing their sense of purpose, connection to others, values, beliefs, and inner peace. Engaging in spiritual activities can have a positive impact on children's physical health by reducing stress, promoting relaxation, and boosting the immune system. Spiritual practices such as meditation, mindfulness, prayer, and gratitude have been shown to lower blood pressure, improve sleep quality, and enhance overall physical resilience. Children's church and fellowship with other Christian kids helps to forge spiritually positive relationships for the future. Additionally, nurturing children's spiritual growth can help them develop a strong sense of identity, self-awareness, and emotional resilience, which are essential for coping with challenges, managing stress, and maintaining mental and emotional well-being. By fostering spiritual growth, children can cultivate qualities such as compassion, empathy, kindness, and moral values that contribute to their social interactions, relationships, and overall happiness. Overall, integrating spiritual practices into children's lives can lead to holistic development, benefiting their physical, mental, emotional, and social well-being in profound ways. What are some of the spiritual activities for your babies? I have listed some examples of activities for you.

Spiritual activities for children

1. Meditation: Introduce children to mindfulness and meditation practices by guiding them through simple breathing exercises or visualization techniques to promote calmness and self-awareness.

2. Nature walks: Take family walks in nature, encouraging children to appreciate the beauty of the outdoors, connect with the environment, and foster a sense of wonder and gratitude.

3. Mindful eating: Practice mindful eating as a family by savoring each bite, expressing gratitude for the food, and encouraging reflection on where the food came from and the effort that went into its production.

4. Reading spiritual stories: Read religious or spiritual stories and parables together as a family to impart moral values, ethical lessons, and teachings of wisdom and compassion.

5. Family prayer or meditation time: Set aside regular time for family prayer, meditation, or reflection to nurture a sense of spirituality, gratitude, and connection with each other and a higher power.

6. Acts of kindness: Engage in acts of service and kindness as a family, such as volunteering at a local charity, helping neighbors in need, or participating in community service projects to instill values of compassion and empathy.

7. Gratitude journaling: Start a family gratitude journal where everyone can write down things, they are thankful for each day, promoting a mindset of positivity, appreciation, and mindfulness.

8. Creation activities: Engage in creative activities like painting, drawing, crafting, or music-making to express spirituality, emotions, and inner thoughts through art.

9. Reflection time: Set aside quiet time for family members to reflect on their day, share their feelings, express gratitude, and set intentions for the future, fostering self-awareness and emotional well-being.

10. Family rituals or traditions: Establish family rituals or traditions that hold spiritual significance, such as lighting candles together, saying prayers before meals, celebrating religious holidays, or participating in ceremonies that promote unity, connection, and shared values.

Engaging in spiritual growth activities as a child and as a family can have profound benefits for overall well-being. Spiritual practices such as meditation, prayer, mindfulness, reflection, and gratitude can help children and families cultivate inner peace, emotional resilience, and a sense of purpose. These activities provide opportunities for self-exploration, personal growth, and connection to something greater than oneself, fostering a deep sense of fulfillment and contentment. Spiritual growth activities can also promote mental well-being by reducing stress, anxiety, and negative emotions, and enhancing emotional regulation, self-awareness, and empathy. Additionally, engaging in spiritual activities as a family can strengthen bonds, improve communication, and create a sense of unity and shared values. By practicing spirituality together, families can support each other's spiritual journeys, instill moral values, and deepen their relationships.

Overall, integrating spiritual growth activities into the lives of children and families can lead to improved mental health, emotional well-being, connectedness, resilience, and a sense of harmony and purpose in life.

The Bible offers guidance and wisdom on the importance of training and disciplining a child. Proverbs 22:6 states, "Train up a child in the way he should go; even when he is old, he will not depart from it." This verse emphasizes the importance of teaching children, moral values, guiding them towards righteousness, and providing them with a strong foundation of faith. Proverbs 29:17 also emphasizes the significance of discipline in child-rearing, stating, "Discipline your son, and he will give you rest; he will give delight to your heart." This verse highlights the positive impact of discipline in shaping a child's behavior and character. Ephesians 6:4 instructs parents to raise their children with love and discipline, stating, "Fathers, do not provoke your children to anger, but bring them up in the discipline and instruction of the Lord." This verse emphasizes the importance of balancing discipline with love and nurturing, ensuring that children are raised with respect for authority, obedience, and a strong spiritual foundation. Couples bonding and keeping the romance alive are vital aspects of a successful and fulfilling relationship. Building a strong bond through communication, shared experiences, and trust fosters emotional intimacy and connection between partners. Additionally, maintaining romance through gestures, quality time, and physical affection helps keep the spark alive and ignites passion in the relationship. By prioritizing these elements, couples can enhance their relationship, strengthen their connection, and create a lasting partnership filled with love and happiness. Deuteronomy 6:6-7 - "These commandments that I give you today are to be on your hearts. Impress them on your children. Talk about them when you sit at home and when you walk along the road, when lie down and when you get up."

- Meaning: In these verses, parents are instructed to pass down the teachings of God to their children continuously. The passage emphasizes the importance of integrating spiritual instruction into everyday life and keeping God's commandments at the forefront of family interactions.

These verses underscore the significance of nurturing, instructing, and guiding children in a loving and God-centered manner, aiming to help them develop a strong moral foundation and faith as they grow.

Empowering kids for a healthy future involves instilling positive habits and promoting overall well-being from a young age. As parents and or guardians, your role is crucial in setting a positive example and creating a supportive environment for your children to thrive. Encouraging healthy habits such as regular exercise, nutritious eating, adequate sleep, and managing stress can have a profound impact on your child's physical and mental health. By prioritizing their well-being and teaching them the importance of self-care, you are equipping them with the tools they need to make healthy choices throughout their lives. Remember, your guidance and support are instrumental in shaping their future health and well-being. By working together to empower kids for a healthy future, we can ensure they have the best chance of leading happy, fulfilling lives.

A family that prioritizes health and wellness cultivates a strong foundation that promotes physical, mental, and emotional growth for all its members. From making nutritious food choices to engaging in regular physical activity and fostering open communication, a family's commitment to a healthy lifestyle can have far-reaching benefits for everyone involved.

1. Promotes Physical Health and Fitness:

Encouraging regular exercise and physical activity as a family not only improves physical health but also strengthens bonds between family members. Activities such as outdoor sports, hiking, biking, or even regular walks together can be enjoyable ways to stay active while spending quality time together. Moreover, preparing home-cooked meals using fresh, wholesome ingredients helps instill healthy eating habits in children from a young age, reducing the risk of obesity and chronic diseases.

2. Enhances Mental and Emotional Well-being:

A supportive and nurturing family environment plays a crucial role in promoting mental and emotional well-being. Open communication, active listening, and creating a safe space for sharing thoughts and feelings foster strong relationships and emotional resilience within the family. Engaging in mindfulness practices, such as meditation or yoga, as a family can also help reduce stress and improve overall mental health.

3. Strengthens Family Bond and Connection:

Prioritizing family health and lifestyle allows for shared experiences and bonding opportunities that create lasting memories and strengthen familial relationships. When family members come together to participate in physical activities, cook meals, or engage in hobbies collectively, they build a sense of camaraderie and togetherness that contributes to a supportive and loving family dynamic.

4. Sets a Positive Example for Children:

Children learn by example, and when parents prioritize their own health and wellness, they set a positive model for their children to follow. Teaching children the importance of self-care, healthy eating, and regular exercise early on instills lifelong habits that contribute to their overall well-being as they grow into adulthood. Family involvement in maintaining health and lifestyle choices reinforces the values of teamwork, responsibility, and mutual support.

5. Fosters Resilience and Adaptability:

Embracing a healthy lifestyle as a family helps build resilience and adaptability in facing life's challenges together. By prioritizing health and wellness, families can navigate stressful situations more effectively, support each other through difficult times, and develop coping mechanisms that promote mental and emotional strength.

A strong family is characterized by various key elements that contribute to its cohesion, resilience, and overall well-being. Here are some factors that contribute to building a strong family, along with explanations of each:

1. Communication:

Open, honest, and respectful communication is essential for building a strong family. Members should feel comfortable expressing their thoughts, feelings, and concerns, and actively listening to one another. Effective communication helps resolve conflicts, build trust, and foster a sense of understanding and connection within the family.

2. Mutual Support:

Strong families provide a supportive environment where members can rely on each other in times of need. Offering emotional, practical, and moral support creates a sense of security and belonging within the family. Being there for one another through challenges and celebrations helps strengthen relationships and promotes unity.

3. Quality Time Together:

Spending quality time together as a family is vital for building strong bonds and creating lasting memories. Engaging in activities, traditions, and shared experiences fosters a sense of connection and closeness among family members. Whether it's family dinners, game nights, outings, or vacations, these shared moments contribute to a sense of unity and belonging.

4. Respect and Empathy:

Respecting each other's opinions, boundaries, and differences is crucial for a strong family dynamic. Empathy and understanding foster compassion and harmony within the family, promoting a culture of kindness, acceptance, and mutual respect. Valuing each family member's unique qualities and perspectives strengthens relationships and builds trust.

5. Clear Roles and Responsibilities:

Establishing clear roles, responsibilities, and expectations within the family helps create a sense of structure and order. When each member knows their role and contribution to the family unit, it promotes cooperation, teamwork, and accountability. Setting boundaries and communicating expectations effectively can help prevent conflicts and misunderstandings.

6. Flexibility and Adaptability:

Strong families are adaptable and resilient in the face of challenges and changes. Being able to adjust to new situations, accept differences, and navigate obstacles together promotes growth and unity. Flexibility in communication, problem-solving, and decision-making allows the family to evolve and thrive through various life transitions.

7. Shared Values and Goals:

Having shared values, beliefs, and goals can unite a family and provide a sense of purpose and direction. When family members align around a common vision or set of principles, it strengthens their bond and fosters a sense of unity. Working towards common objectives and supporting each other's aspirations cultivates a strong sense of family identity and cohesion.

In summary, prioritizing family health and lifestyle is essential for creating a harmonious and thriving family unit. By making conscious choices to prioritize physical health, mental well-being, and emotional connections, families can lay a strong foundation for overall happiness and fulfillment. Embracing a healthy lifestyle together not only benefits individual family members but also strengthens the bonds that hold the family together, fostering a sense of unity, support, and love that last. Also, a strong family is built on a foundation of communication, support, quality time, respect, clear roles, adaptability, and shared values. By prioritizing these key elements and nurturing positive relationships within the family unit, members can cultivate a strong sense of unity, cohesion, and resilience that withstands challenges and strengthens bonds over time.

It starts with you and ends with you; your efforts will produce your results.

Reflecting on the one-year journey and celebrating achievements

Reflecting on a One-Year Wellness Journey and Celebrating Achievements: A Call to Action

Dear Reader,

As you journey through the ups and downs of life, it is essential to take a moment to pause, reflect, and celebrate the milestones you have achieved along the way. One profound way to do this is by reflecting on your one-year wellness journey and acknowledging the growth and progress you have made in your pursuit of a healthier, happier life.

Embarking on a wellness journey is not merely about physical fitness or weight loss – it is about holistic well-being that encompasses all aspects of your being: physical, mental, emotional, and spiritual. By dedicating time and effort to nurture yourself in these areas, you are investing in your long-term health and happiness.

Begin by setting aside some quiet moments to reflect on the past year. Consider the goals you set for yourself, the challenges you faced, and the victories you achieved. Take stock of the changes you have made – whether it be adopting a more balanced diet, committing to a regular exercise routine, prioritizing self-care, or seeking support for your mental and emotional well-being.

Celebrate the small wins – the days you chose a nourishing meal over fast food, the mornings you woke up early to do yoga, the moments you practiced gratitude and mindfulness. These seemingly insignificant actions are building blocks towards a healthier, more fulfilling life. Acknowledge the progress you have made, no matter how small, and give yourself credit for the effort you have put in.

It is important to also recognize the setbacks and challenges you may have faced along the way. Life is not always smooth sailing, and there will inevitably be obstacles that test your resolve and commitment to your wellness journey. Reflect on these moments with compassion and curiosity – what lessons have they taught you? How can you use them as opportunities for growth and learning?

As you reflect on your one-year wellness journey, remember to celebrate your achievements – both big and small. Whether it is reaching a fitness milestone, breaking a harmful habit, or experiencing a shift in mindset, every step forward is worth honoring. Celebrate yourself, for the progress you have made, the resilience you have shown, and the dedication you have demonstrated towards your well-being.

I urge you, dear reader, to take the time to reflect on your one-year wellness journey and celebrate the achievements that have brought you to this moment. Embrace the journey with gratitude and humility and use it as a springboard for continued growth and transformation. Your well-being is a precious gift – cherish it, nurture it, and celebrate it every step of the way.

With warmest regards,

Toni Williams

Guidance on how to maintain a wellness-centered lifestyle beyond the book.

"One Year Wellness Journey" is a powerful guide that will empower you and your loved ones to embrace their own wellness journeys and transform their lives for the better. Through this book, you will gain the knowledge, motivation, and practical tools necessary to make lasting positive changes and achieve holistic well-being. In the quest for a wellness-centered lifestyle that goes beyond the pages of a book, it is essential to cultivate habits and practices that support long-term health, happiness, and fulfillment for both you and your family. Building upon the foundation laid by the knowledge and inspiration gleaned from your reading, here are some practical guidance and strategies to help you maintain a wellness-centered lifestyle for the long haul:

1. Consistency is Key: One of the most important aspects of maintaining a wellness-centered lifestyle is consistency. Make a commitment to prioritize your well-being every day, whether it's through healthy eating, regular exercise, mindfulness practices, or self-care routines. Consistency is the key to creating lasting positive change and reaping the benefits of a healthy lifestyle over time.

2. Set Realistic Goals: When it comes to maintaining wellness, setting realistic and achievable goals is crucial. Break down larger goals into smaller, manageable steps that you can work towards each day. Celebrate your progress along the way and adjust your goals as needed to stay motivated and on track.

3. Establish Healthy Habits: Incorporate healthy habits into your daily routine that support your overall well-being. This might include meal planning and prepping, scheduling regular exercise sessions, practicing mindfulness or meditation, getting enough sleep,

and staying hydrated. These habits will not only benefit you but also create a culture of wellness within your family.

4. Prioritize Self-Care: Self-care is a vital component of maintaining a wellness-centered lifestyle. Make time for activities that nourish your body, mind, and soul, whether it's reading a book, taking a relaxing bath, spending time in nature, or connecting with loved ones. Encourage your family members to prioritize self-care as well, fostering a culture of well-being and balance within your household.

5. Stay Connected: Building a strong support network is essential for maintaining a wellness-centered lifestyle. Stay connected with friends, family, or a community of like-minded individuals who can provide encouragement, accountability, and inspiration on your wellness journey. Share your goals and challenges with others and offer support in return to create a culture of mutual growth and support.

6. Practice Gratitude: Cultivating a practice of gratitude can have profound effects on your overall well-being. Take time each day to reflect on the things you are grateful for, whether it's a beautiful sunset, a kind gesture from a loved one, or a moment of quiet reflection. Encourage your family members to join you in practicing gratitude, fostering a positive and appreciative mindset within your household.

7. Adapt and Evolve: Wellness is a journey, not a destination, and it's important to remain flexible and open to growth and change along the way. Be willing to adapt your routines, goals, and practices as needed to better align with your evolving needs and aspirations. Embrace new challenges and opportunities for growth, and approach them with curiosity and an open heart.

In conclusion, maintaining a wellness-centered lifestyle beyond the confines of a book requires dedication, intention, and a commitment to care and personal growth. By incorporating these strategies into your daily life and fostering a culture of well-being within your family, you can create a sustainable, fulfilling lifestyle that supports your overall health and happiness for years to come. Embrace the journey with openness and enthusiasm, knowing that the path to wellness is a continuous evolution of self-discovery and empowerment for both you and your loved ones.

Men, Women, and Children's Health Tips

In this helpful section, we will explore valuable health tips tailored specifically for men, women, and children. Each demographic has unique health considerations and priorities that are essential to address to promote overall well-being and longevity.

Women's Tips

Ladies! As a woman, I believe that health tips play a crucial role in empowering women to prioritize their well-being and lead healthier lives. Women juggle multiple responsibilities and often put the needs of others before their own, making it essential to focus on self-care and healthy habits. By implementing practical and sustainable health tips tailored to women's unique needs, they can enhance their physical, mental, and emotional health. Some key healthy tips for women include:

1. Prioritize regular physical activity, such as aerobic exercises, strength training, and yoga, to improve cardiovascular health, maintain muscle tone, and reduce stress.

2. Consume a nutrient-rich diet with plenty of fruits, vegetables, whole grains, lean proteins, and healthy fats to support energy levels, immune function, and overall health.

3. Stay hydrated by drinking an adequate amount of water daily to promote digestion, metabolism, and skin health.

4. Practice self-care rituals such as mindfulness, meditation, deep breathing exercises, or journaling to reduce stress levels and enhance mental well-being.

5. Get regular health check-ups, screenings, and preventive care to monitor hormone levels, bone health, and overall wellness.

6. Ensure an adequate intake of calcium and vitamin D to support bone health and reduce the risk of osteoporosis.

7. Prioritize sleep hygiene by establishing a relaxing bedtime routine and aiming for 7-9 hours of quality sleep each night to promote restorative rest.

By embracing these health tips and making them a part of their daily routine, women can take charge of their health and well-being, leading to a healthier, happier, and more fulfilling life.

Healthy Ladies Let's Get It! Here is a detailed list of healthcare visit tips for women's health:

1. Schedule regular well-woman exams with a gynecologist or healthcare provider to monitor your overall health, reproductive health, and screen for any potential health issues.

2. Prioritize preventative care, such as cervical cancer screenings (Pap smears), breast cancer screenings (mammograms), and other recommended screenings based on your age and risk factors.

3. Prepare for healthcare visits by making a list of any symptoms, concerns, or questions you have about your health to discuss with your provider.

4. Keep track of your menstrual cycles, any changes in your menstrual patterns, and any other potential factors that may impact your reproductive health.

5. Be proactive about discussing your family medical history, including any hereditary conditions, with your healthcare provider to assess your risk for certain health issues.

6. Advocate for your health by seeking clarification on any recommendations made by your healthcare provider, asking about potential treatment options, and expressing any concerns you may have.

7. Stay up to date on vaccinations and other preventative measures to protect your health, such as the HPV vaccine for cervical cancer prevention.

8. Follow through with any recommended follow-up care, screenings, or referrals to specialists, if necessary, to address any health concerns identified during your healthcare visit.

9. Practice self-care and prioritize your mental health by seeking support when needed, practicing mindfulness, and engaging in activities that promote well-being.

By following these healthcare visit tips, women can take an active role in their health and well-being, ensuring they receive the necessary care and screenings to maintain optimal health throughout their lives.

We don't often discuss cleaning the vagina and maybe it's a touchy subject or just between mother or guardian and daughter back in the day. Believe it or not some girls didn't receive this needed information. So, no matter the reason, let's get it in here. Using a vaginal douche, or vaginal irrigation, is a practice of rinsing the vagina with water or a mixture of fluids for hygienic or therapeutic purposes. *However, it is important to note that regular douching is not recommended by healthcare professionals as it can disrupt the natural balance of the vagina and increase the risk of infections and other complications.* If you are considering using a vaginal douche, it is important to follow these detailed tips for proper use:

1. Consult with a Healthcare Provider:

- Before using a vaginal douche, consult with your healthcare provider to discuss whether it is necessary or safe for your individual situation.

2. Choose the Right Product:

- If your healthcare provider recommends using a vaginal douche, select a commercially prepared, pre-packaged solution specifically designed for vaginal douching.

- Avoid homemade douching solutions, as they may contain ingredients that can irritate or disrupt the vaginal pH balance.

3. Follow Instructions Carefully:

- Read and follow the instructions provided on the packaging of the vaginal douche carefully.

- Pay attention to the recommended amount of solutions to use and proper technique for administration.

4. Maintain Hygiene:

- Wash your hands thoroughly before and after using a vaginal douche to prevent the introduction of harmful bacteria into the vagina.

5. Use Lukewarm Water:

- Use lukewarm water for vaginal douching to avoid causing discomfort or irritation, as water that is too hot or too cold can be harsh on the vaginal tissues.

6. Gentle Administration:

- Administer the douche gently and slowly to avoid discomfort or causing injury to the delicate vaginal tissues.

- Do not use excessive pressure when flushing the vagina.

7. Practice Moderation:

- Limit the frequency of vaginal douching to only when recommended by a healthcare provider and avoid regular or routine use.

- Overuse of vaginal douches can disrupt the natural balance of vaginal flora and increase the risk of infections.

8. Avoid Scented Products:

- Avoid using scented vaginal douches or products, as fragrances and chemicals can lead to irritation and allergic reactions in the vaginal area.

9. Stop if Discomfort Occurs:

- Discontinue using a vaginal douche if you experience any discomfort, pain, itching, burning, or unusual discharge after douching.

- Consult your healthcare provider if you have any concerns or adverse reactions.

10. Focus on Overall Vaginal Health:

- Instead of relying on vaginal douches for hygiene, prioritize overall vaginal health through regular gentle cleansing with mild soap and water, wearing breathable underwear, and maintaining good hygiene practices.

It is important to remember that vaginal douching is generally not necessary for vaginal health and can do more harm than good. If you have concerns about vaginal odor, discharge, or infections, it is best to consult with a healthcare provider for proper diagnosis and treatment recommendations.

Tampons

Using tampons safely and correctly is essential for maintaining vaginal health and preventing complications. Here is a detailed list of tips for the proper use of tampons for women:

1. Choose the Right Absorbency:

- Select tampons with the appropriate absorbency level for your menstrual flow, opting for a lower absorbency tampon on lighter days and a higher absorbency tampon on heavier days.

- Avoid using tampons with a higher absorbency level than needed to reduce the risk of Toxic Shock Syndrome (TSS).

2. Wash Your Hands:

- Before inserting a tampon, wash your hands with soap and water to reduce the risk of introducing harmful bacteria into the vaginal canal.

3. Use Applicator or Digital Tampons:

- Choose between tampons with applicators or digital tampons, based on your personal preference for insertion.

- Follow the instructions provided on the tampon packaging for proper insertion.

4. Positioning:

- Find a comfortable position for inserting the tampon, such as sitting on the toilet, standing with one leg elevated, or squatting.

- Relax your pelvic muscles to make insertion easier and more comfortable.

5. Insertion:

- Hold the tampon applicator or tampon with clean hands and gently insert it into the vaginal opening at a slight angle towards the small of your back.

- Push the tampon all the way into the vagina until your fingers or the applicator touches the opening.

6. Comfortable Fit:

- Ensure the tampon is inserted far enough into the vagina to feel comfortable and secure without causing discomfort or being felt.

- The tampon string should hang outside the vaginal opening for easy removal later.

7. Change Regularly:

- Change tampons every 4 to 8 hours, depending on the flow of your period, to prevent bacterial overgrowth and reduce the risk of TSS.

- Avoid leaving a tampon in for longer than 8 hours.

8. Remove and Discard Carefully:

- To remove the tampon, gently pull the string at the base of the tampon until it comes out.

- Wrap the used tampon in toilet paper and dispose of it in a sanitary disposal unit or trash can. Do not flush tampons down the toilet.

9. Be Mindful of String Position:

- Be cautious when using tampons with applicators to ensure the string does not get caught in the applicator during insertion.

- Check that the tampon is properly inserted, and the string is positioned outside the vagina before discarding the applicator.

10. Know the Signs of TSS:

- Educate yourself about the symptoms of Toxic Shock Syndrome, such as sudden high fever, rash resembling sunburn, dizziness, and vomiting.

- Seek medical attention immediately if you experience any symptoms of TSS while using tampons.

Following these tips for the proper use of tampons can help ensure a comfortable and safe experience during menstruation. It is always essential to listen to your body, follow the instructions provided by the tampon manufacturer, and consult with a healthcare provider if you have any concerns or experience discomfort while using tampons.

Using menstrual pads correctly is important for maintaining hygiene and comfort during menstruation. Here is a detailed list of tips for the proper use of menstrual pads for women:

1. Choose the Right Absorbency:

- Select menstrual pads with the appropriate absorbency level for your flow intensity, choosing heavier pads for heavy flow days and lighter pads for lighter flow days.

- Avoid using pads with a higher absorbency level than needed to prevent skin irritation and discomfort.

2. Change Regularly:

- Change your menstrual pad every 3-4 hours, or more frequently if needed, to maintain cleanliness and prevent odors.

- Avoid wearing a pad for longer than 8 hours to reduce the risk of bacterial growth and skin irritation.

3. Wash Your Hands:

- Before and after changing your menstrual pad, wash your hands thoroughly with soap and water to reduce the risk of introducing harmful bacteria to the vaginal area.

4. Proper Placement:

- Attach the adhesive side of the pad to the inside of your underwear, ensuring it is centered and positioned correctly to absorb menstrual flow effectively.

- Make sure the pad securely adheres to your underwear to prevent shifting or leaks.

5. Comfortable Fit:

- Ensure the pad is comfortable and fits snugly against your body without causing chafing or irritation.

- Opt for pads with soft, breathable materials to increase comfort and reduce the risk of skin sensitivity.

6. Dispose Properly:

- After removing a used pad, fold it and wrap it securely in its wrapper or toilet paper before disposing of it in a waste bin.

- Avoid flushing menstrual pads down the toilet, as they can clog plumbing systems and harm the environment.

7. Maintain Hygiene:

- Change your pad immediately if it becomes soaked or saturated to prevent leaks and maintain optimal hygiene during menstruation.

- Use intimate wipes or a gentle cleanser to clean the vaginal area before applying a fresh pad if access to water is limited.

8. Avoid Fragrances:

- Choose unscented menstrual pads to reduce the risk of skin irritation, allergic reactions, and disruption of the natural pH balance of the vagina.

- Fragrance-free pads are gentler on sensitive skin and less likely to cause discomfort.

9. Storage and Disposal:

- Store your menstrual pads in a cool, dry place to prevent moisture buildup and maintain their integrity.

- Keep a supply of pads on hand, especially during your menstrual cycle, to ensure you are prepared for changes and unexpected flow.

10. Track Your Cycle:

- Keep track of your menstrual cycle using a calendar, app, or journal to anticipate the start of your period and make sure you have an adequate supply of pads available.

- Monitoring your cycle can help you stay prepared and manage your menstrual hygiene effectively.

By following these detailed tips for the proper use of menstrual pads, you can ensure a comfortable and hygienic experience during your menstrual cycle. It is essential to prioritize your comfort, hygiene, and overall well-being while managing your period. If you have concerns about menstrual pad usage or experience any discomfort, consult with a healthcare provider for guidance and support.

Maxi pads

If your like some women like me who don't prefer to use tampons, pads are the next option. Using menstrual pads correctly is important for maintaining hygiene and comfort during menstruation. Here is a detailed list of tips for the proper use of menstrual pads for women:

1. Choose the Right Absorbency:

- Select menstrual pads with the appropriate absorbency level for your flow intensity, choosing heavier pads for heavy flow days and lighter pads for lighter flow days.

- Avoid using pads with a higher absorbency level than needed to prevent skin irritation and discomfort.

2. Change Regularly:

- Change your menstrual pad every 3-4 hours, or more frequently if needed, to maintain cleanliness and prevent odors.

- Avoid wearing a pad for longer than 8 hours to reduce the risk of bacterial growth and skin irritation.

3. Wash Your Hands:

- Before and after changing your menstrual pad, wash your hands thoroughly with soap and water to reduce the risk of introducing harmful bacteria to the vaginal area.

4. Proper Placement:

- Attach the adhesive side of the pad to the inside of your underwear, ensuring it is centered and positioned correctly to absorb menstrual flow effectively.

- Make sure the pad securely adheres to your underwear to prevent shifting or leaks.

5. Comfortable Fit:

- Ensure the pad is comfortable and fits snugly against your body without causing chafing or irritation.

- Opt for pads with soft, breathable materials to increase comfort and reduce the risk of skin sensitivity.

6. Dispose Properly:

- After removing a used pad, fold it and wrap it securely in its wrapper or toilet paper before disposing of it in a waste bin.

- Avoid flushing menstrual pads down the toilet, as they can clog plumbing systems and harm the environment.

7. Maintain Hygiene:

- Change your pad immediately if it becomes soaked or saturated to prevent leaks and maintain optimal hygiene during menstruation.

- Use intimate wipes or a gentle cleanser to clean the vaginal area before applying a fresh pad if access to water is limited.

8. Avoid Fragrances:

- Choose unscented menstrual pads to reduce the risk of skin irritation, allergic reactions, and disruption of the natural pH balance of the vagina.

- Fragrance-free pads are gentler on sensitive skin and less likely to cause discomfort.

9. Storage and Disposal:

- Store your menstrual pads in a cool, dry place to prevent moisture buildup and maintain their integrity.

- Keep a supply of pads on hand, especially during your menstrual cycle, to ensure you are prepared for changes and unexpected flow.

10. Track Your Cycle:

- Keep track of your menstrual cycle using a calendar, app, or journal to anticipate the start of your period and make sure you have an adequate supply of pads available.

- Monitoring your cycle can help you stay prepared and manage your menstrual hygiene effectively.

By following these detailed tips for the proper use of menstrual pads, you can ensure a comfortable and hygienic experience during your menstrual cycle. It is essential to prioritize your comfort, hygiene, and overall well-being while managing your period. If you have concerns about menstrual pad usage or experience any discomfort, consult with a healthcare provider for guidance and support.

A self-breast exam

A self-breast exam is an important part of a woman's overall health routine as it can help in the early detection of any breast changes or abnormalities. Here is a detailed summary and step-by-step guide on how to perform a self-breast exam:

1. Timing: It is recommended for women to perform a breast self-exam once a month. The best time to do a breast self-exam is a few days after your period ends when your breasts are less likely to be swollen or tender.

2. Visual Inspection:

- Stand in front of a mirror with your hands on your hips.

- Look for any changes in the size, shape, or contour of your breasts, as well as any skin dimpling, swelling, or redness.

- Check for any nipple discharge or inversion.

3. In the Shower:

- Raise one arm and use the opposite hand to examine the corresponding breast.

- Use the pads of your fingers to feel for any lumps or thickening in your breast tissue.

- Make sure to cover the entire breast and armpit area in a circular motion.

4. Lying Down:

- Lie down on a flat surface and place a pillow under your right shoulder.

- Use your left hand to examine your right breast using the same circular motion with the pads of your fingers.

- Repeat the process for the left breast using your right hand.

5. Underarm Area:

- Check the underarm area for any lumps or swelling as breast tissue can extend into the armpit.

6. Repeat Regularly:

- Get into the habit of performing breast self-exams every month to become familiar with the normal look and feel of your breasts.

It is important to note that while self-breast exams can help in the early detection of breast changes, they are not a substitute for regular mammograms and clinical breast exams by a healthcare provider. If you notice any changes in your breasts during a self-exam, it is important to consult a healthcare professional for further evaluation.

Remember, early detection is key in the successful treatment of breast cancer.

Women have different types of breast tissue, each with its own characteristics and functions. Understanding the composition of breast tissue can help women become more aware of their breast health and any changes that may occur. Here is a detailed summary and list of the different types of breast tissue for women:

1. Glandular Tissue:

- Glandular tissue is also known as the functional tissue of the breast.

- It is responsible for producing milk and comprises lobes, lobules, and ducts.

- Lobules contain milk-producing glands, while ducts are responsible for carrying milk to the nipple during breastfeeding.

2. Fibrous Tissue:

- Fibrous tissue provides structure and support to the breast.

- It includes connective tissue, ligaments, and collagen fibers that help maintain the shape and firmness of the breast.

3. Adipose Tissue:

- Adipose tissue, or fatty tissue, is the main component of the breast.

- It provides cushioning and protection to the breast tissue.

- The amount of adipose tissue in the breast varies among individuals and can affect breast size and density.

4. Suspensory Ligaments:

- Suspensory ligaments are fibrous bands that help support and position the breast tissue.

- Changes in these ligaments can affect breast shape and can contribute to conditions like breast ptosis (sagging).

5. Breast Lobes:

- The breast is divided into several lobes, each containing lobules that produce milk.

- The number of lobes can vary among individuals and can affect milk production and breast health.

Understanding the different types of breast tissue and their functions can help women become more knowledgeable about their breast health. Changes in breast tissue, such as lumps, pain, or thickening, should be promptly evaluated by a healthcare provider to rule out any underlying issues. Regular breast self-exams, clinical breast exams, and mammograms can help in the early detection of any abnormalities or changes in breast tissue.

Caring for your breasts is an important aspect of overall health and well-being for women. Here is a detailed summary and list of tips on how to take care of your breasts:

1. Wearing the Right Bra:

- Choose a supportive and properly fitted bra to provide adequate support and reduce strain on your breast tissue.

- Avoid wearing bras that are too tight or have underwires that can constrict blood flow.

2. Maintain a Healthy Weight:

- Maintain a healthy weight through a balanced diet and regular exercise.

- Excess weight can lead to increased breast size and density, which may affect breast health.

3. Regular Exercise:

- Engage in regular physical activity to promote overall health and lower the risk of breast cancer.

- Exercise can help improve circulation, reduce inflammation, and maintain breast tissue health.

4. Breast Self-Exams:

- Perform monthly breast self-exams to become familiar with the normal look and feel of your breasts.

- Check for any changes, lumps, or abnormalities during self-exams and consult a healthcare provider if you notice any concerns.

5. Healthy Diet:

- Maintain a balanced diet rich in fruits, vegetables, whole grains, lean proteins, and healthy fats.

- Consuming a nutritious diet can help support overall health, including breast health.

6. Limit Alcohol Consumption:

- Limit alcohol intake as excessive drinking has been linked to an increased risk of breast cancer.

- Moderation is key when it comes to alcohol consumption for breast health.

7. Avoid Smoking:

- Quit smoking or avoid exposure to secondhand smoke.

- Smoking is associated with an increased risk of breast cancer and other health issues.

8. Regular Health Check-ups:

- Schedule regular clinical breast exams and mammograms as recommended by your healthcare provider.

- Early detection through screenings can help in the timely diagnosis and treatment of breast-related issues.

9. Sun Protection:

- Protect your breasts from harmful UV rays by applying sunscreen or covering up when spending time outdoors.

- Prolonged sun exposure can lead to skin damage and potentially increase the risk of skin cancer.

Taking care of your breasts involves a combination of self-care practices, healthy lifestyle choices, and regular screening. By incorporating these tips into your routine, you can promote breast health and overall well-being. Remember that any concerns or changes in your breasts should be discussed with a healthcare provider for proper evaluation and management.

Taking care of your bras and ensuring proper bra fit are important for maintaining breast health and comfort. Here is a detailed summary and list of tips for women about bras and their health:

1. Bra Fit:

- The key to comfort and breast health is wearing a bra that fits properly.

- Get professionally fitted for a bra to ensure the right band and cup size.

- Bras that are too tight or too loose can lead to discomfort, chafing, and even breathing difficulties.

2. Avoiding Underwires:

- Underwires can dig into breast tissue, causing discomfort and potentially impacting breast health.

- Choose the wireless bras or bras with flexible underwire that provides support without digging into the skin.

3. Bra Maintenance:

- Wash your bras regularly to keep them clean and hygienic.

- Hand wash bras or use a lingerie bag when machine washing to protect delicate fabrics.

- Air dry bras to maintain their shape and elasticity.

4. Rotate Your Bras:

- Avoid wearing the same bra consecutively to allow the elastic to rest and regain its shape.

- Rotate between different bras to extend their lifespan and provide adequate support.

5. Sports Bras:

- Invest in a good quality sports bra for physical activities to reduce breast movement and strain on breast tissue.

- Choose a sports bra that offers proper support and compression based on your activity level.

6. Bra Straps:

- Adjust bra straps to ensure they are not digging into your shoulders or causing discomfort.

- Straps should provide support without leaving marks on your skin.

7. Bra Material:

- Choose bras made from breathable, moisture-wicking fabrics to avoid skin irritation and promote airflow.

- Avoid bras with rough seams or fabrics that can chafe or irritate sensitive skin.

8. Bra Shopping:

- Regularly reassess your bra size as it can change due to weight fluctuations, pregnancy, or aging.

- Invest in bras that provide adequate support and coverage for your breast size and shape.

9. Bra-Free Time:

- Give your breasts a break by going bra-free, when possible, especially at home or while sleeping.

- Allowing your breast tissue to relax without constriction can promote circulation and lymphatic flow.

10. Listen to Your Body:

- Pay attention to how your bras feel throughout the day and adjust them if you experience discomfort.

- Consult a bra fitting specialist or healthcare provider if you have concerns about your bra fit or breast health.

By following these tips, you can ensure that your bras provide the necessary support, comfort, and care for your breast health. Prioritizing proper bra fit and maintenance can contribute to overall breast health and well-being.

Knowing when to replace aging bras is important for maintaining proper support, comfort, and breast health. Here is a detailed list of tips on when to throw away your aging bras:

1. Loss of Elasticity:

- Bras lose elasticity over time due to regular wear and washing.

- Replace bras when the elastic band no longer provides firm support around your ribcage.

2. Visible Wear and Tear:

- Check your bras for signs of wear such as fraying, stretching, or fabric damage.

- Discard bras with visible wear and tear that compromise their structural integrity.

3. Faded or Discolored:

- Bras that have lost their color or appear faded may indicate age and frequent washing.

- Replace bras that look worn out or discolored, as it can affect their support and appearance.

4. Protruding Underwires:

- Underwires that poke out or become misshapen can be uncomfortable and may cause skin irritation.

- Discard bras with protruding underwires to avoid discomfort and potential injury.

5. Loose Straps:

- Bra straps can stretch out over time, leading to them slipping off your shoulders or causing discomfort.

- Replace bras with loose or stretched-out straps that no longer provide adequate support.

6. Changes in Breast Size:

- Weight fluctuations, hormonal changes, pregnancy, or aging can alter your breast size and shape.

- Evaluate your bras regularly and replace them if they no longer fit properly or offer adequate support.

7. Stretched Out Cups:

- Bras with stretched out or misshapen cups may no longer provide the desired lift or coverage.

- Replace bras with stretched out cups to maintain proper breast support and shape.

8. Redness or Irritation:

- Bras that cause redness, irritation, or rubbing against your skin may indicate poor fit or fabric quality.

- Discard bras that cause discomfort or skin issues to prevent further irritation.

9. Lack of Comfort:

- If your bras no longer feel comfortable or supportive, it may be time to replace them.

- Listen to your body and replace bras that no longer provide the desired level of comfort and fit.

10. Recommended Lifespan:

- While the lifespan of a bra can vary depending on quality and care, on average, bras should be replaced every 6-12 months.

- Regularly assess the condition of your bras and replace them as needed to ensure proper support and comfort. When it's time don't fight it, toss it!

By monitoring the condition of your bras and recognizing these signs of aging, you can maintain optimal breast health and comfort by replacing bras when necessary. Prioritize proper bra fit and support to ensure the well-being of your breasts. If it has safety pins, repeated sew tracks or tape of some sort, or if it's a breastfeeding bra and your child is a teen or adult; throw it out.

Taking care of your shoes is important not just for the longevity of your footwear but also for the health of your feet, posture, and overall well-being. Here is a detailed summary and list of tips for women about their shoes and their health:

1. Proper Shoe Fit:

- Ensure that your shoes fit properly with enough room in the toe box to prevent crowding and discomfort.

- Avoid shoes that are too tight or too loose, as they can lead to foot pain, blisters, and other foot problems.

2. Supportive Footwear:

- Choose shoes with adequate arch support and cushioning to provide stability and reduce the risk of foot injuries.

- Consider orthotic inserts or custom-made insoles for additional support if needed.

3. Rotate Your Shoes:

- Rotate between different pairs of shoes to prevent excessive wear on a particular pair and allow time for shoes to air out and dry.

- Wearing the same shoes every day can lead to increased wear and tear and potential foot issues.

4. Comfort Over Fashion:

- Prioritize comfort when selecting shoes over style, especially for everyday footwear.

- Look for shoes that are comfortable, provide proper support, and are suitable for the activity you will be engaging in.

5. Replace Worn-Out Shoes:

- Check your shoes regularly for signs of wear such as worn-out soles, heel erosion, or decreased support.

- Replace shoes that show visible signs of wear to prevent foot pain, discomfort, and potential foot conditions.

6. Proper Shoe Care:

- Clean your shoes regularly to remove dirt, dust, and bacteria that can accumulate inside and cause foot odor.

- Use appropriate cleaning products based on the material of your shoes and follow care instructions provided by the manufacturer.

7. Appropriate Shoe Selection:

- Choose footwear suited to the activity you will be doing, whether it's walking, running, hiking, or working.

- Wear shoes with good traction and support for physical activities to prevent slips, falls, and injuries.

8. Lace-Up and Secure Shoes:

- Ensure that your shoes are securely fastened and laced up properly to provide stability and prevent foot and ankle injuries.

- Avoid wearing shoes that are too loose or slip off easily, as they can impact your gait and posture.

9. Check for Proper Alignment:

- Pay attention to how your shoes affect your posture and gait.

- Choose shoes that promote proper alignment of the feet, ankles, knees, and back to reduce the risk of musculoskeletal issues.

10. Listen to Your Feet:

- Pay attention to any discomfort, pain, or changes in your feet when wearing certain shoes.

- If you experience foot pain or discomfort, consider consulting a podiatrist or footwear specialist for advice on proper shoe selection and foot health.

In following these tips and prioritizing the health of your feet through proper shoe selection and care, you can prevent foot problems, enhance comfort, and promote overall well-being.

Remember that the right shoes play a crucial role in supporting your feet and maintaining your mobility and comfort throughout the day.

Knowing when to replace aging shoes is essential for maintaining foot health, preventing discomfort, and ensuring proper support. Here is a detailed list of tips on when to throw away your aging shoes as a woman:

1. Worn-Out Soles:

- Check the bottom of your shoes for visible signs of wear, such as worn-down treads or smooth surfaces.

- Replace shoes with worn-out soles to prevent slips, loss of traction, and potential foot injuries.

2. Loss of Cushioning:

- Over time, the cushioning and padding inside shoes can compress and lose their ability to provide adequate shock absorption.

- Discard shoes with flattened or worn-out cushioning to prevent foot fatigue, pain, and impact-related injuries.

3. Visible Damage:

- Examine your shoes for visible damage, such as tears, holes, or peeling materials.

- Replace shoes with visible damage that compromises their structural integrity and may lead to discomfort or injuries.

4. Uneven Wear Patterns:

- Pay attention to any uneven wear patterns on the soles or heels of your shoes.

- Shoes that show uneven wear may indicate biomechanical issues or improper fit, leading to foot discomfort and potential foot problems.

5. Lack of Support:

- If you notice a decrease in support, stability, or structure in your shoes, it may be time to replace them.

- Shoes that no longer provide adequate support can contribute to foot strain, arch pain, or misalignment issues.

6. Odor and Bacteria:

- Persistent foot odor or visible signs of bacteria growth inside shoes may indicate poor ventilation and hygiene.

- Replace shoes with lingering odors or bacterial growth to prevent foot infections, fungal issues, and skin irritations.

7. Discomfort or Pain:

- Listen to your feet and pay attention to any discomfort, pain, or irritation when wearing your shoes.

- If you experience persistent foot pain or discomfort, it may be time to replace your shoes with more supportive and comfortable options.

8. Outdated Style:

- While style is not the primary factor in determining shoe health, outdated or out-of-fashion shoes may indicate that it's time for an update.

- Update your shoe wardrobe with current styles that meet your fashion preferences and support your foot health.

9. Beyond Repair:

- Shoes that are beyond repair, with irreparable damage or structural issues, should be discarded.

- Attempting to continue wearing shoes that cannot be fixed may lead to further foot problems and discomfort.

10. Recommended Lifespan:

- Depending on the frequency of wear, activity level, and shoe quality, most shoes have a lifespan of 300-500 miles or 6-12 months.

- Regularly assess the condition of your shoes and replace them as needed to maintain foot health and comfort. If you know they have seen better days, toss them; let it go.

Through recognizing these signs of aging in your shoes and knowing when to replace them, you can ensure proper foot support, comfort, and overall foot health as a woman. Prioritize the well-being of your feet by investing in quality footwear and replacing aging shoes in a timely manner.

Men's Health Tips

As a wife, I understand the importance of prioritizing men's health and wellness. Men often face unique challenges when it comes to maintaining good health, but by incorporating simple yet effective health tips into their daily routines, they can improve their overall well-being and longevity. From making smart dietary choices to staying active and managing stress, there are several key tips that can positively impact men's health:

1. Eat a balanced diet rich in fruits, vegetables, whole grains, lean proteins, and healthy fats to support overall health.

2. Engage in regular physical activity, such as strength training, cardiovascular exercise, and flexibility work, to promote cardiovascular health, muscle strength, and flexibility.

3. Stay hydrated by drinking an adequate amount of water throughout the day.

4. Get regular health screenings and check-ups to monitor blood pressure, cholesterol levels, and other key health indicators.

5. Practice stress management techniques such as mindfulness, meditation, or relaxation exercises to reduce stress levels and support mental well-being.

6. Prioritize adequate sleep by establishing a consistent sleep routine and aiming for 7-9 hours of quality sleep per night.

7. Limit alcohol consumption and avoid smoking or using tobacco products to reduce the risk of chronic diseases and improve overall health.

By using these healthy tips into their daily lives, men can take proactive steps toward maintaining their health and well-being, ultimately leading to a happier and more fulfilling life.

Alright fellas! Here is a detailed list of healthcare visit tips for men's health:

1. Schedule regular check-ups with a primary care physician or healthcare provider to monitor your overall health and address any concerns or potential health issues.

2. Prioritize preventative care, such as blood pressure screenings, cholesterol screenings, and recommended cancer screenings, based on your age and risk factors.

3. Discuss any family medical history with your healthcare provider to understand your potential risk for certain conditions and diseases.

4. Bring a list of any symptoms, concerns, or questions you have about your health to your healthcare visit to ensure you address them with your provider.

5. Stay informed about your weight, diet, exercise habits, and any lifestyle factors that may impact your health, and be open to discussing them with your healthcare provider.

6. Be proactive about discussing mental health concerns or stressors with your healthcare provider, as mental health is an important component of overall well-being.

7. Follow through with any recommended follow-up care, screenings, or referrals to specialists, if needed, to address any health issues identified during your healthcare visit.

8. Advocate for your health by seeking information on treatment options, clarifying any recommendations made by your healthcare provider, and expressing any worries you may have.

9. Stay up to date on vaccinations and other preventative measures recommended for men's health, such as the flu vaccine and the HPV vaccine.

With these healthcare visit tips, men can prioritize their health and well-being, ensuring they receive the necessary care, screenings, and support to maintain optimal health throughout their lives.

Physical Fitness

Maintaining a healthy level of physical fitness is crucial for men to support overall health, reduce the risk of chronic diseases, and improve quality of life. Here are detailed tips focusing on cardiovascular and strength training exercises tailored specifically for men:

Cardiovascular Exercise Tips:

1. Start Slowly: If you are new to cardiovascular exercise, begin with low-impact activities such as walking, cycling, or swimming to gradually build endurance.

2. Consult a Healthcare Provider: Before starting a new exercise regimen, especially if you have existing health conditions, consult with your healthcare provider to ensure safety.

3. Set Realistic Goals: Establish achievable fitness goals for your cardiovascular workouts, such as increasing duration, intensity, or frequency gradually over time.

4. Mix It Up: Incorporate a variety of cardio exercises into your routine to keep it interesting and target different muscle groups effectively.

5. Monitor Intensity: Pay attention to your heart rate during cardio workouts and aim to reach a moderate intensity level for optimal cardiovascular benefits.

Strength Training Tips:

1. Proper Form: Focus on maintaining proper form during strength training exercises to prevent injuries and maximize results.

2. Progressive Overload: Gradually increase the resistance or weight used in strength training to continuously challenge your muscles and promote growth.

3. Include Compound Exercises: Incorporate compound movements such as squats, deadlifts, and bench presses into your routine for efficient muscle recruitment and overall strength development.

4. Rest and Recovery: Allow adequate rest days between strength training sessions to give your muscles time to repair and grow stronger.

5. Nutrition: Ensure you are consuming enough protein and essential nutrients to support muscle recovery and growth after strength training workouts.

Additional Tips for Overall Fitness:

1. *Consistency*: Aim for regularity in your workout routine, whether it's cardio or strength training, to maintain progress and see results.

2. *Warm-Up and Cool Down:* Prioritize warming up before exercise to prepare your muscles and joints for exercise, and cooling down afterward to help with muscle recovery, reduce muscle soreness, and flexibility.

3. *Proper Form*: Focus on using correct form during exercises to prevent injuries and maximize the effectiveness of your workout. Consider working with a trainer to learn proper techniques.

4. *Listen to Your Body*: Pay attention to your body's signals and adjust your workouts as needed

to prevent overtraining or injury. If you experience pain or discomfort, stop, and consult with a healthcare professional.

5. *Gradual Progression*: Avoid pushing yourself too hard too soon. Gradually increase the intensity, duration, or weight of your workouts to prevent overtraining and injury.

6. *Hydration*: Stay properly hydrated before, during, and after exercise to support optimal performance and recovery.

7. *Professional Guidance*: Consider working with a certified personal trainer to develop a tailored fitness plan and ensure proper technique in your workouts.

8. *Rest and Recovery*: Give your body time to rest and recover between workouts to allow your muscles to repair and grow stronger. Adequate rest is essential for overall performance and injury prevention.

9. *Mix It Up*: Incorporate a variety of exercises, including strength training, cardiovascular activities, and flexibility exercises, to target different muscle groups and prevent boredom.

Remember to tailor your workout routine to your individual fitness level, goals, and any underlying health conditions. Consulting with a fitness professional can help you create a safe and effective workout plan that meets your needs.

Via including these detailed men's health tips on cardiovascular and strength training into your fitness routine, you can improve fitness levels, enhance overall health, and achieve your wellness goals effectively. Remember to prioritize safety, consistency, and proper technique in your workouts for long-term success.

Now we also must work out the best from our body. Here is a sample 3-day workout plan. Please note that this plan can be adjusted based on individual fitness level, goals, and preferences:

Three-day weekly plan

Day 1: Full Body Strength Training

1. Warm-Up: 5-10 minutes of light cardio (e.g., jogging, jumping jacks)

2. Squats: 3 sets of 12 reps

3. Push-Ups: 3 sets of 10 reps

4. Bent-Over Rows: 3 sets of 12 reps

5. Lunges: 3 sets of 10 reps per leg

6. Plank: 3 sets of 30 seconds

7. Cool Down: Stretching exercises for the major muscle groups

Day 2: Cardio and Core

1. Warm-Up: 5-10 minutes of dynamic stretching

2. Running or Cycling: 20-30 minutes of moderate-intensity cardio

3. Russian Twists: 3 sets of 15 reps (each side)

4. Bicycle Crunches: 3 sets of 20 reps

5. Mountain Climbers: 3 sets of 20 reps (each leg)

6. Plank with Side Leg Raises: 3 sets of 12 reps (each side)

7. Cool Down: Stretching exercises for the core and lower body

Day 3: Upper Body Strength and Cardio

1. Warm-Up: 5-10 minutes of light cardio

2. Bench Press: 3 sets of 10 reps

3. Pull-Ups or Lat Pulldowns: 3 sets of 10 reps

4. Shoulder Press: 3 sets of 12 reps

5. Bicep Curls: 3 sets of 12 reps

6. Triceps Dips: 3 sets of 10 reps

7. Jump Rope: 10 minutes of high-intensity intervals

8. Cool Down: Stretching exercises for the upper body

Remember to listen to your body, stay hydrated, and adjust the intensity of the workouts based on your individual fitness level. Don't overdo it trying to be superman. Take it easy on yourself in the beginning and adjust. It's also important to incorporate rest days into your routine to allow for proper recovery and muscle growth. If you're new to exercise or have any health concerns, consider consulting with a fitness professional before starting a new workout plan.

Maintaining healthy testosterone levels

Maintaining healthy testosterone levels is crucial for men's overall health, vitality, and well-being. Here are some specific men's health tips to help improve and support healthy testosterone levels:

1. Regular Exercise: Engage in regular physical activity, including both cardiovascular exercise and weight training. Exercise has been shown to boost testosterone levels, especially high-intensity interval training (HIIT) and strength training exercises like squats, deadlifts, and bench presses.

2. Manage Stress: Chronic stress can contribute to lower testosterone levels. Practice stress-reducing techniques such as meditation, deep breathing exercises, yoga, or mindfulness to help lower stress hormones like cortisol and support healthy testosterone production.

3. Get Sufficient Sleep: Aim for 7-9 hours of quality sleep each night. Lack of sleep can disrupt hormone production, including testosterone. Create a relaxing bedtime routine and ensure your sleep environment is conducive to restful sleep.

4. Healthy Diet: Maintain a balanced diet rich in nutrient-dense foods. Include plenty of lean proteins, healthy fats (such as omega-3 fatty acids), whole grains, fruits, and vegetables. Foods high in zinc, vitamin D, and magnesium can also support healthy testosterone levels.

5. Maintain Healthy Weight: Excess body fat can contribute to lower testosterone levels. Aim to maintain a healthy weight through a combination of regular exercise and a balanced diet.

6. Limit Alcohol Intake: Excessive alcohol consumption can negatively impact testosterone levels. Limit your intake of alcohol, especially binge drinking, to support optimal hormone balance.

7. Stay Hydrated: Dehydration can affect hormone production and overall health. Drink an adequate amount of water throughout the day to support optimal bodily functions, including hormone regulation.

8. Avoid Endocrine Disruptors: Reduce exposure to chemicals found in plastics, pesticides, and personal care products that can disrupt hormone balance. Look for natural and organic products whenever possible.

9. Consider Testosterone-Boosting Supplements: Some men may benefit from natural supplements that support testosterone production, such as vitamin D, zinc, D-aspartic acid, and fenugreek extract. Consult with a healthcare provider before starting any new supplement regimen.

10. Regular Health Check-ups: Schedule routine visits with your healthcare provider to monitor testosterone levels and address any concerns or symptoms of low testosterone, such as decreased libido, fatigue, or changes in mood.

It's important to remember that individual hormone levels can vary, and if you suspect you have low testosterone or are experiencing symptoms of hormonal imbalance, it's best to consult with a healthcare provider for an accurate diagnosis and personalized treatment plan.

Prostate Health

Look guys I know this is the one topic your comfort level drops off at and you really don't like talking about, but this is an important subject. The prostate is a small gland located below the bladder in men that plays a crucial role in the reproductive system. It produces fluid that nourishes and protects sperm, helping them survive in the acidic environment of the vagina. Maintaining prostate health is essential for overall well-being and can help prevent conditions such as prostatitis, benign prostatic hyperplasia (BPH), and prostate cancer.

Here are some men's health tips to support prostate health and make it easier to manage:

1. Maintain a Healthy Diet: Eating a balanced diet rich in fruits, vegetables, whole grains, lean proteins, and healthy fats can support overall prostate health. Include foods high in antioxidants, such as tomatoes, berries, and green leafy vegetables, as they can help reduce inflammation and protect the prostate.

2. Stay Active: Regular physical activity and exercise can help support prostate health and reduce the risk of prostate conditions. Aim for at least one hundred and fifty minutes of moderate intensity exercise each week, such as brisk walking, cycling, or swimming.

3. Maintain a Healthy Weight: Excess body weight, especially around the waist, has been linked to an increased risk of prostate conditions. Maintain a healthy weight through a combination of regular exercise and a balanced diet.

4. Hydrate Properly: Adequate hydration is crucial for prostate health. Drink plenty of water throughout the day to help flush out toxins and support proper prostate function.

5. Limit Alcohol and Caffeine: Excessive consumption of alcohol and caffeine can irritate the prostate gland. Limit your intake of these substances to help maintain prostate health.

6. Quit Smoking: Smoking has been linked to an increased risk of prostate cancer and other prostate conditions. If you smoke, consider quitting to reduce your risk and improve overall health.

7. Practice Safe Sex: Engaging in safe sex practices can help reduce the risk of sexually transmitted infections that can affect prostate

health. Use condoms to protect against infections and maintain overall sexual health.

8. Regular Prostate Screenings: Men over the age of 50 (or earlier if at higher risk) should consider regular prostate screenings, including a prostate-specific antigen (PSA) blood test and a digital rectal exam. Early detection of prostate conditions can lead to more effective treatment.

9. Manage Stress: Chronic stress can negatively impact prostate health. Practice stress-reducing techniques such as meditation, deep breathing exercises, yoga, or mindfulness to help lower stress levels and support overall well-being.

10. Consult Your Healthcare Provider: If you experience any symptoms of prostate issues, such as frequent urination, difficulty urinating, blood in urine or semen, or pelvic pain, consult your healthcare provider for evaluation and appropriate management.

By following these men's health tips and taking proactive steps to support prostate health, you can reduce the risk of prostate conditions and maintain overall well-being. Prioritizing regular screenings and maintaining a healthy lifestyle can help you support your prostate health for years to come.

Making examination easier

Men I understand that this examination is mentally and physically uncomfortable but, there are ways to make it a bit easier to tolerate and get done. Prostate examinations, including digital rectal exams (DRE) and prostate-specific antigen (PSA) tests, are important for early detection and monitoring of prostate conditions, such as prostate cancer. While these examinations may cause discomfort or anxiety for some men, there are steps you can take to make the process easier and more comfortable:

1. Choose a Trusted Healthcare Provider: Select a healthcare provider whom you feel comfortable with and trust. Open communication with your provider can help alleviate any concerns or fears you may have about the examination.

2. Communicate Your Concerns: Before the examination begins, talk to your healthcare provider about any fears or anxieties you have regarding the procedure. They can provide you with information about what to expect and offer reassurance.

3. Relaxation Techniques: Practice relaxation techniques, such as deep breathing exercises or visualization, to help calm your nerves before and during the examination. Relaxing your body and mind can make the process more comfortable.

4. Ask Questions: If you have any questions about the examination, don't hesitate to ask your healthcare provider. Understanding the

purpose of the examination and how it will be conducted can help ease your nerves.

5. Positioning: During a DRE, your healthcare provider will have you bend over a table or lie on your side with your knees drawn up towards your chest. Finding a comfortable position and communicating any discomfort during the examination can make the process easier.

6. Gentle Approach: A skilled healthcare provider will perform the examination with care and sensitivity. If you experience pain or discomfort during the examination, inform your provider immediately so adjustments can be made.

7. Distraction Techniques: Engage in distraction techniques, such as focusing on your breathing, counting numbers, or visualizing a calming scene, to take your mind off the discomfort during the examination.

8. Use Lubrication: Lubrication is typically used during a DRE to reduce friction and discomfort. If you find the sensation uncomfortable, don't hesitate to ask your healthcare provider to apply more lubrication.

9. Positive Reinforcement: Remind yourself of the importance of the much-needed examination in detecting and preventing serious health conditions. Positive reinforcement can help motivate you to undergo the examination even if it causes some discomfort.

10. Follow-Up Care: After the examination, discuss the results with your healthcare provider and follow any recommendations for further testing or monitoring. Regular prostate check-ups are essential for maintaining optimal prostate health.

By employing these men's health tips and strategies, you can make prostate examinations easier and more manageable. Guys, you are important to the ladies, your families, and friends so your health matters. Remember that early detection of prostate conditions can lead to better treatment outcomes and improved overall health.

Sexual Health

Maintaining sexual health is an important aspect of overall well-being for men. Sexual health encompasses various factors, including erectile function, stamina, libido, and overall sexual satisfaction. Here are some detailed men's health tips to promote sexual health, enhance erections, and improve stamina:

1. Maintain a Healthy Lifestyle:

- Eat a balanced diet rich in fruits, vegetables, whole grains, lean proteins, and healthy fats to support overall health and circulation.

- Stay physically active to improve cardiovascular health, blood flow, and overall stamina.

- Maintain a healthy weight to reduce the risk of obesity and associated sexual health issues.

2. Manage Stress:

- Chronic stress can negatively impact sexual health and erectile function. Practice stress-reducing techniques such as meditation, yoga, deep breathing exercises, or mindfulness.

- Engage in regular physical activity to release endorphins and reduce stress levels.

3. Quit Smoking:

- Smoking can constrict blood vessels and impair blood flow, leading to erectile dysfunction. Quitting smoking can improve circulation and overall sexual health.

4. Limit Alcohol Intake:

- Excessive alcohol consumption can impact sexual performance and reduce libido. Drink alcohol in moderation to support sexual health and function.

5. Stay Hydrated:

- Proper hydration is essential for overall health, including sexual health and stamina. Drink an adequate amount of water each day to stay hydrated.

6. Get Sufficient Sleep:

- Lack of sleep can affect hormone levels, including testosterone, and impact sexual health. Aim for 7-9 hours of quality sleep each night to support optimal sexual function.

7. Communicate with Your Spouse:

- Open communication with your partner about sexual desires, preferences, and concerns can improve intimacy and sexual satisfaction.

- Discuss any difficulties or issues with erectile function or stamina with your partner to reduce anxiety and enhance mutual understanding.

8. Explore Different Sexual Techniques:

- Experimenting with different sexual techniques, positions, and activities can help maintain interest and excitement in the bedroom.

- Focus on pleasure and intimacy rather than performance alone.

9. Consult a Healthcare Provider:

- If you experience persistent issues with erectile dysfunction, low libido, or stamina, speak with a healthcare provider for a proper evaluation and personalized treatment plan.

- Your healthcare provider may recommend medications, therapies, or lifestyle modifications to address sexual health concerns.

10. Pelvic Floor Exercises:

- Kegel exercises can strengthen the pelvic floor muscles, improve blood flow to the genital area, and enhance erectile function and stamina.

- Learn how to perform Kegel exercises and incorporate them into your routine to support sexual health.

By selecting and encompassing these men's health tips into your lifestyle and prioritizing sexual health, you can enhance erectile function, improve stamina, and promote overall well-being in the realm of sexual wellness. Remember that seeking guidance from healthcare professionals is crucial for addressing any underlying issues and optimizing your sexual health.

Erectile dysfunction (ED)

This is another touchy topic but one we must discuss. After all it is a piece of your healthy journey and it's ok you are not alone, there is hope and help. Erectile dysfunction (ED) is a common condition that can impact men's sexual health and overall quality of life. Here are some detailed men's health tips on erectile dysfunction, along with management strategies to address this issue:

Men's Health Tips for Erectile Dysfunction:

1. Healthy Lifestyle Habits:

- Maintain a healthy diet rich in fruits, vegetables, whole grains, lean proteins, and healthy fats to support overall health and circulation.

- Stay physically active through regular exercise to improve cardiovascular health and blood flow, which are essential for erectile function.

2. Manage Chronic Health Conditions:

- Control underlying health conditions such as diabetes, high blood pressure, and high cholesterol, as they can contribute to erectile dysfunction.

- Work with your healthcare provider to manage these conditions effectively and minimize their impact on sexual health.

3. Quit Smoking and Limit Alcohol Intake:

- Smoking can restrict blood flow to the penis and contribute to erectile dysfunction. Quitting smoking can improve circulation and sexual health.

- Limit alcohol consumption, as excessive drinking can affect sexual performance and libido.

4. Maintain a Healthy Weight:

- Excess body weight can lead to hormonal imbalances and reduce testosterone levels, affecting erectile function. Maintain a healthy weight through diet and exercise.

5. Reduce Stress and Anxiety:

- Stress and anxiety can contribute to erectile dysfunction. Practice stress-reducing techniques such as meditation, deep breathing exercises, or therapy to manage stress levels.

- Engage in relaxation activities to promote mental well-being and reduce performance anxiety related to sexual activity.

Management Strategies for Erectile Dysfunction:

1. Medications:

- Discuss with your healthcare provider the use of medications such as sildenafil (Viagra), tadalafil (Cialis), or vardenafil (Levitra) to help improve erectile function.

- These medications work by increasing blood flow to the penis and can be effective in treating erectile dysfunction.

2. Counseling and Therapy:

- Consider seeking therapy or counseling to address psychological factors contributing to erectile dysfunction, such as performance anxiety, relationship issues, or stress.

- Couples therapy can be beneficial in improving communication and intimacy in relationships affected by ED.

3. Vacuum Erection Devices:

- Vacuum erection devices are non-invasive devices that help draw blood into the penis to create an erection. They can be used as a temporary solution for erectile dysfunction.

4. Penile Injections or Urethral Suppositories:

- In some cases, medications can be injected into the penis or inserted into the urethra to help achieve an erection.

- These treatments can be effective for men who do not respond to oral medications.

5. Penile Implants:

- In severe cases of erectile dysfunction that do not respond to other treatments, penile implants can be surgically implanted to allow for an erection.

- Discuss the risks and benefits of this procedure with a urologist or healthcare provider.

6. Lifestyle Modifications:

- Incorporate regular exercise, a healthy diet, and stress-reducing activities into your daily routine to support overall health and sexual function.

- Avoid excessive alcohol consumption, quit smoking, and maintain a healthy weight to improve erectile function.

Remember, erectile dysfunction is a common condition that is treatable, and seeking help from a healthcare provider is important for an accurate diagnosis and personalized treatment plan. By incorporating these men's health tips and management strategies into your routine, you can address erectile dysfunction and improve your sexual health and well-being.

For men facing erectile dysfunction, it is important to remember that you are not alone in dealing with this common and treatable condition. Seeking help and taking steps to address erectile dysfunction is a proactive and courageous decision that can lead to improved sexual health and overall well-being. Remember that erectile dysfunction does not define your masculinity or worth as a person. With the right support, guidance, and treatment options available, there is hope for improving your sexual function and regaining confidence in intimate situations. By seeking help from healthcare professionals, making lifestyle changes, and exploring treatment options, you are taking control of your health and prioritizing your well-being. Stay positive, stay hopeful, and know that there are resources and solutions available to help you on your journey towards better sexual health. You deserve to feel empowered, supported, and encouraged as you navigate this aspect of your men's health journey.

Andropause (male menopause)

Men do not go through menopause; instead, they may experience andropause, often referred to as male menopause, which involves a gradual decline in testosterone levels as they age. Here are some men's health tips on managing symptoms related to declining libido and hormonal changes in men:

Men's Health Tips for Managing Andropause Symptoms and Libido Health:

1. Healthy Diet and Exercise:

- Maintain a balanced diet rich in fruits, vegetables, lean proteins, whole grains, and healthy fats to support overall health and hormone balance.

- Engage in regular physical activity, including both cardiovascular exercise and strength training, to boost energy levels, improve circulation, and support hormone production.

2. Stress Management:

- Practice stress-reducing techniques such as meditation, deep breathing exercises, yoga, or mindfulness to lower cortisol levels and promote hormonal balance.

- Prioritize self-care activities that help you relax and unwind, such as hobbies, spending time in nature, or listening to music.

3. Quality Sleep:

- Aim for 7-9 hours of quality sleep each night to support hormone regulation, energy levels, and overall well-being.

- Establish a bedtime routine and create a restful sleep environment to promote restorative sleep.

4. Regular Health Check-ups:

- Schedule routine visits with your healthcare provider to monitor hormone levels, discuss symptoms, and explore treatment options.

- Consider requesting hormone level tests to assess testosterone and other hormone levels.

5. Communication and Support:

- Openly communicate with your partner about any changes in libido or sexual function and work together to find solutions that meet both of your needs.

- Seek support from a healthcare provider, therapist, or support group to address any emotional or relationship challenges related to andropause.

6. Hormone Therapy and Medications:

- Discuss with a healthcare provider the potential benefits and risks of hormone replacement therapy or medications to address testosterone deficiency and improve libido.

- Follow your healthcare provider's recommendations for monitoring hormone levels and adjusting treatment as needed.

7. Lifestyle Modifications:

- Limit alcohol consumption and avoid smoking, as these habits can negatively impact hormone levels and libido.

- Manage weight through a healthy diet and regular exercise to support hormonal balance and overall health.

In incorporating these men's health tips for managing andropause symptoms and supporting libido health, you can proactively address changes related to hormonal shifts and maintain optimal well-being as you age. Remember that seeking guidance from healthcare professionals is essential for evaluating symptoms, developing a personalized treatment plan, and optimizing your health during the andropause transition.

Andropause Symptoms

Andropause, also known as male menopause, refers to the natural decline in testosterone levels that occurs in men as they age. This hormonal transition, like menopause in women, can bring about a range of symptoms that may impact physical, emotional, and sexual health. Here is a detailed description of common andropause symptoms:

1. Decreased Libido: One of the hallmark symptoms of andropause is a decrease in sex drive or libido. Reduced testosterone levels can affect sexual desire and performance, leading to changes in sexual activity and satisfaction.

2. Erectile Dysfunction: Changes in testosterone levels can contribute to difficulties achieving or maintaining an erection, resulting in erectile dysfunction. This can impact sexual function and influence self-esteem and confidence.

3. Fatigue and Reduced Energy: Men experiencing andropause may notice a decline in energy levels and increased fatigue, even with adequate rest. This fatigue can affect daily activities and motivation.

4. Loss of Muscle Mass: Lower testosterone levels can lead to a decrease in muscle mass and strength, making it more challenging to maintain muscle tone and overall physical strength.

5. Increased Body Fat: Andropause can result in changes in body composition, including an increase in body fat, particularly around the abdomen. This change in fat distribution can also contribute to metabolic issues and an increased risk of chronic conditions.

6. Mood Changes: Hormonal fluctuations during andropause can impact mood stability and emotional well-being. Men may experience irritability, mood swings, anxiety, or depression as a symptom of these hormonal changes.

7. Sleep Disturbances: Some men going through andropause may experience disruptions in sleep patterns, including difficulty falling asleep, staying asleep, or experiencing restful sleep. Poor sleep quality can further exacerbate fatigue and mood disturbances.

8. Memory and Cognitive Changes: Hormonal fluctuations during andropause can affect cognitive function, memory, and concentration. Men may notice lapses in memory, cognitive fog, or difficulty focusing on tasks.

9. Hot Flashes: While less common in men than in women, some men may experience hot flashes or night sweats during andropause because of hormonal changes.

10. Decreased Bone Density: Lower testosterone levels can contribute to reduced bone density, increasing the risk of osteoporosis and fractures in men going through andropause.

It's essential to note that the presence and severity of andropause symptoms can vary from one individual to another, and some men may experience few or no noticeable symptoms. If you suspect you are experiencing symptoms of andropause, it is advisable to consult with a healthcare provider for a proper diagnosis and personalized management plan tailored to your specific needs.

Maintaining Feet Health

Yes, fellas' healthy feet are important also. Maintaining good foot health is essential for overall well-being, mobility, and comfort. Here are some detailed men's health tips on feet health, along with strategies for management:

Tips for Maintaining Feet Health:

1. Proper Footwear:

- Wear shoes that fit well and provide adequate support for your feet. Avoid shoes that are too tight, narrow, or have high heels.

- Choose shoes with good arch support and cushioning to reduce pressure on the feet and prevent common foot problems.

2. Regular Foot Care:

- Wash your feet daily with warm water and mild soap, paying special attention to areas between the toes.

- Trim toenails straight across to prevent ingrown nails and maintain good foot hygiene.

- Moisturize your feet regularly to prevent dry, cracked skin.

3. Foot Exercises:

- Perform simple foot exercises, such as toe curls, ankle circles, and stretching exercises, to improve flexibility and strengthen the muscles in your feet.

- Roll a tennis ball or frozen water bottle under your feet to massage and relieve tension.

4. Maintain a Healthy Weight:

- Excess body weight can put added pressure on your feet and contribute to foot pain and conditions such as plantar fasciitis and flat feet.

- Maintain a healthy weight through a balanced diet and regular exercise to reduce strain on your feet.

5. Monitor Foot Health:

- Check your feet regularly for signs of redness, swelling, sores, blisters, or any other unusual changes.

- Be mindful of any pain, numbness, or tingling in your feet, as these could be signs of underlying health issues.

Management Strategies for Common Foot Problems:

1. Plantar Fasciitis:

- If you experience heel pain, particularly in the morning or after prolonged standing, consider using orthotic inserts or heel cups to support your arches.

- Stretch your calves and plantar fascia regularly to help alleviate pain and improve flexibility.

2. Athlete's Foot:

- Keep your feet clean and dry, especially between the toes, to prevent fungal infections.

- Use antifungal powders or creams to treat and prevent athlete's foot.

3. Blisters and Calluses:

- Wear properly fitting shoes to reduce friction and prevent blisters.

- Use padding or moleskin to protect areas prone to blisters and calluses. If a blister develops, avoid popping it to prevent infection.

4. Ingrown Toenails:

- Trim toenails straight across to prevent ingrown nails. If you develop an ingrown toenail, soak your foot in warm water and gently lift the edge of the nail away from the skin.

- Seek professional care from a podiatrist if an ingrown toenail becomes infected or painful.

5. Heel Spurs:

- Apply ice to reduce inflammation and pain in the heel area.

- Stretch your calf muscles and plantar fascia regularly to alleviate stress on the heels.

By following these men's health tips for feet health and implementing management strategies for common foot problems, you can maintain healthy and happy feet for improved mobility and overall well-being. If you experience persistent foot pain or have concerns about your foot health, consult a healthcare provider or a podiatrist for proper evaluation and treatment.

Here is a detailed summary and list of tips about feet health, shoes, and when to throw them away for men:

Summary:

Feet health is essential for overall well-being, and wearing the right shoes plays a crucial role in maintaining healthy feet. Men should pay attention to the fit, support, and quality of their shoes to prevent foot problems such as blisters, calluses, and even more serious conditions like plantar fasciitis. Knowing when to replace old shoes is also important to avoid discomfort and potential foot injuries.

Tips for Feet Health and Shoes for Men:

1. Choose the right shoe size: Make sure your shoes fit properly with enough room for your toes to move comfortably without being too tight or too loose.

2. Search for good arch support: Look for shoes that provide adequate arch support to prevent conditions like flat feet or plantar fasciitis.

3. Quality over quantity: Invest in high-quality shoes made of breathable materials that offer cushioning and support for your feet.

4. Rotate your shoes: Avoid wearing the same pair of shoes every day to allow them to air out and prevent odor and bacteria buildup.

5. Keep your shoes clean: Regularly clean your shoes to prevent dirt and bacteria from accumulating, which can cause foot infections.

6. Replace worn-out shoes: Pay attention to signs of wear and tear such as worn-out soles, flattened cushioning, or visible damage, and replace your shoes when needed.

7. Listen to your feet: If you experience discomfort, pain, or notice any changes in your feet while wearing certain shoes, consider switching to a more suitable pair.

When to Throw Away Old Shoes:

1. When the soles are worn out and offer little to no traction.

2. When the cushioning is flattened and no longer provides adequate support.

3. When the shoes show visible signs of damage such as holes, tears, or cracks.

4. When you experience foot pain or discomfort while wearing the shoes, it indicates they no longer offer proper support.

5. When the shoes have a persistent odor that cannot be eliminated even after cleaning.

By adhering to these tips and knowing when to replace old shoes, men can maintain good feet health and prevent foot problems in the long run.

Foot fungus

The stinky truth is you don't like it, your family may complain about it and it may even be embarrassing at times but it's okay, there is help. Here is a detailed summary and list of tips about foot fungus, shoes, symptoms, treatment, and when to throw them away for men:

Summary:

Foot fungus, also known as athlete's foot, is a common fungal infection that can affect men's feet. It thrives in warm, moist environments like sweaty shoes and can cause symptoms such as itching, redness, peeling skin, and a foul odor. Proper foot hygiene, wearing breathable shoes, and knowing when to replace old shoes are essential in preventing and managing foot fungus in men.

Tips for Dealing with Foot Fungus and Shoes for Men:

1. Keep feet clean and dry: Wash your feet daily with soap and water, and make sure to thoroughly dry them, especially between the toes, to prevent fungal growth.

2. Wear moisture-wicking socks: Choose socks made of breathable materials like cotton or moisture-wicking fabrics to keep your feet dry and reduce the risk of fungus growth.

3. Rotate your shoes: Avoid wearing the same pair of shoes every day to allow them to air out and prevent moisture buildup that can contribute to foot fungus.

4. Choose breathable shoes: Opt for shoes made of breathable materials like leather or mesh to promote air circulation and reduce sweat accumulation.

5. Treat shoes with antifungal spray: Use antifungal sprays or powders inside your shoes to help kill fungus and prevent its spread.

6. Avoid sharing shoes: Do not share shoes with others to reduce the risk of spreading fungal infections.

7. Seek medical treatment: If you suspect you have foot fungus, consult a healthcare professional for proper diagnosis and treatment, which may include antifungal creams or oral medications.

Symptoms of Foot Fungus:

1. Itching and burning sensation on the feet.

2. Redness and inflammation of the skin, especially between the toes.

3. Peeling, cracking, or flaking skin on the feet.

4. Foul odor coming from the feet.

5. Blisters or sores on the affected area.

When to Throw Away Old Shoes:

1. If you have been diagnosed with foot fungus, consider discarding shoes that may be harboring the fungus to prevent reinfection.

2. If despite cleaning and treatment, the shoes continue to have a persistent odor or show signs of fungal growth.

3. If the shoes are old, worn out, and no longer provide adequate support and protection for your feet.

By following these tips and being aware of the symptoms of foot fungus, men can take proactive steps to prevent, manage, and treat this common foot condition while also ensuring the health of their feet and shoes.

Children's Tips

Embarking on a journey of cultivating good health habits in children is a noble endeavor with far-reaching benefits. By introducing and reinforcing healthy practices early on, parents and caregivers play a pivotal role in shaping children's overall well-being. To promote optimal health in children, it is essential to prioritize a nutrient-rich diet that includes a colorful array of fruits, vegetables, whole grains, and lean proteins. Encouraging regular physical activity not only strengthens their bodies but also fosters a positive attitude towards staying active throughout their lives. Limiting screen time and promoting outdoor play can help maintain a healthy balance and reduce the risk of sedentary-related health issues. Emphasizing the importance of proper hydration and setting consistent sleep routines are also crucial components of children's health. Additionally, teaching children good hygiene practices, such as regular handwashing and dental care, instills habits that can safeguard their health in the long run. By incorporating these holistic health tips into the lives of children, we empower them to thrive and embrace a lifetime of well-being.

Here is a detailed list of healthy tips for children's health:

1. Encourage a balanced diet rich in fruits, vegetables, whole grains, and lean proteins to ensure they receive essential nutrients for growth and development.

2. Limit sugary snacks and drinks to prevent dental issues, obesity, and other health issues related to excess sugar intake.

3. Promote regular physical activity to strengthen their bones and muscles, improve cardiovascular health, and support overall well-being.

4. Set limits on screen time and encourage outdoor play to reduce sedentary behavior and promote active lifestyles.

5. Ensure they get enough quality sleep each night to support proper growth, cognitive development, and overall health.

6. Teach good hygiene practices, such as regular handwashing, to prevent the spread of illnesses and maintain good health.

7. Schedule regular check-ups with healthcare providers to monitor their growth, development, and address any health concerns early on.

8. Foster open communication about emotions and mental well-being to support their mental health and resilience.

9. Lead by example by incorporating healthy habits into your own lifestyle, showing children the importance of prioritizing their health.

By incorporating these healthy tips into children's daily routines, we can help them establish lifelong habits that promote optimal health and well-being.

Here is a detailed list of tips for children's learning and education for better health:

1. Encourage Active Learning: Incorporate interactive and hands-on learning activities to engage children and promote physical activity. This could include educational games, outdoor exploration, and creative projects.

2. Provide Nutritious Meals: Ensure that children have access to balanced and nutritious meals to support their physical health and cognitive development. Offer a variety of fruits, vegetables, whole grains, and lean proteins in their diet.

3. Promote Regular Physical Activity: Encourage children to engage in regular physical activity to support their overall health and well-being. This could include activities such as sports, dance, yoga, or simply playing outside.

4. Establish Healthy Sleep Habits: Help children develop good sleep habits by establishing a consistent bedtime routine and ensuring they get enough rest each night. A well-rested child is better able to focus and learn.

5. Limit Screen Time: Set limits on screen time for children to promote physical activity, social interaction, and cognitive development. Encourage them to engage in other activities such as reading, arts and crafts, or playing with toys.

6. Provide a Safe and Supportive Environment: Create a safe and supportive learning environment for children that promotes their physical and emotional well-being. This includes ensuring a clean and organized space, offering positive reinforcement, and addressing any concerns they may have.

7. Encourage Social Interaction: Foster opportunities for children to interact with their peers and develop social skills. Social interaction is important for emotional health, empathy, and communication skills.

8. Support Mental Health: Be attentive to children's emotional well-being and provide support when needed. Encourage open communication, teach coping strategies, and seek professional help if necessary.

9. Encourage Lifelong Learning: Instill a love for learning in children by encouraging curiosity, exploration, and a growth mindset. Help them see the value of education for their future health and success.

10. Lead by Example: Model healthy behaviors and habits for children to emulate. Demonstrate the importance of a balanced diet, regular exercise, good sleep, and lifelong learning in your own life.

By following these tips, you can help children develop healthy habits and achieve better health outcomes through education and learning.

Here I have laid out a detailed list of healthcare visit tips for children's health:

1. Schedule regular well-child check-ups with a pediatrician or healthcare provider to monitor your child's growth, development, and overall health.

2. Prioritize preventative care, such as vaccinations and screenings, to protect your child from common childhood illnesses and detect any potential health issues early on.

3. Prepare for healthcare visits by writing down any questions or concerns you have about your child's health and development.

4. Bring your child's medical history, including any medications they are taking, allergies, and relevant family medical history, to share with the healthcare provider.

5. Be an advocate for your child's health by asking questions, seeking clarification, and expressing any worries or uncertainties during the healthcare visit.

6. Follow the healthcare provider's recommendations for follow-up care, screenings, and referrals to specialists, if needed, to ensure your child receives comprehensive and appropriate healthcare.

7. Keep a record of your child's healthcare visits, including notes from the provider, test results, and any recommendations for future care.

8. Promote a positive and open dialogue between your child and their healthcare provider, encouraging them to voice any concerns or questions they may have.

9. Stay informed about age-appropriate milestones and healthcare guidelines for children, so you can advocate for the best possible care for your child.

By following these healthcare visit tips, parents and caregivers can help ensure that their children receive high-quality healthcare and support their overall health and well-being.

When meeting with your child's primary care physician, it is important to ask relevant questions to address your child's health and well-being. Here is a detailed list of questions you may consider asking:

1. What is my child's current growth and development status?

2. Are there any developmental milestones my child should be meeting?

3. What vaccinations does my child need, and are they up to date?

4. Are there any dietary or nutritional recommendations for my child?

5. How can I encourage healthy eating habits and physical activity for my child?

6. Are there any specific health concerns I should be aware of for my child's age?

7. What are the potential risks of common childhood illnesses and how can I prevent them?

8. Are there any screenings or tests my child should undergo at this age?

9. How can I support my child's mental and emotional well-being?

10. Are there any signs or symptoms I should watch for that may indicate a health issue?

11. Can you provide guidance on managing common childhood ailments like colds, fevers, or allergies?

12. Are there any safety considerations or injury prevention tips I should be aware of?

13. How can I establish a good bedtime routine and promote healthy sleep habits for my child?

14. What are the recommendations for screen time and technology use for my child's age group?

15. Are there any resources or educational materials you can provide to support my child's health and development?

Feel free to adjust and add any additional questions based on your child's unique needs and medical history to ensure that you have a comprehensive understanding of your child's health and well-being.

When taking your child to see an optometrist for an eye examination or vision-related concerns, it is important to ask relevant questions to ensure that you are well-informed about your child's eye health. Here is a detailed list of questions you may consider asking your child's optometrist:

1. What is my child's current vision prescription and does my child need glasses or contact lenses?

2. Are there any signs of vision problems that I should be aware of in my child?

3. How often should my child have their eyes examined for optimal eye health and vision correction?

4. Are there any specific eye conditions or diseases that run in our family that could affect my child's eye health?

5. Can you assess my child's eye alignment, focusing abilities, and eye teaming skills to ensure proper visual development?

6. Are there any potential risks or warning signs of vision problems that I should watch for in my child?

7. How can I help my child maintain good eye health and prevent vision issues in the future?

8. Are there any dietary recommendations or supplements that can benefit my child's eye health and vision development?

9. Can you provide tips for managing screen time and digital device use to prevent eye strain in children?

10. Are there any specific activities or exercises that can help improve my child's vision or eye coordination?

11. How can I ensure that my child's school environment is eye-friendly and supportive of good vision health?

12. Can you explain any test results or findings from my child's eye examination in a way that is easy to understand?

13. Are there any concerns or questions my child has about their vision that we should discuss?

14. What treatment options are available if my child is diagnosed with a vision problem, and what are the potential risks or side effects?

15. Are there any recommendations for protecting my child's eyes during sports, outdoor activities, or other recreational pursuits?

Feel free to add any specific questions related to your child's individual eye health concerns, school performance, or any signs of eye discomfort to ensure that your child's eye care needs are fully addressed during the appointment with the optometrist.

General Tips

Asking questions to your healthcare providers is an essential part of receiving quality healthcare and being an active participant in your own health management. Don't be afraid to ask questions.

When meeting with your primary care physician, it's important to ask relevant questions to address your health concerns and make informed decisions regarding your care. Here is a detailed list of questions you may consider asking your primary care physician:

1. What is the nature of my condition/diagnosis?

2. What are the potential causes of my symptoms?

3. What treatment options are available, and which do you recommend?

4. Are there any lifestyle changes I can make to improve my condition?

5. What are the potential side effects of the prescribed treatment?

6. How long will it take for the treatment to show results?

7. Should I follow up with you for a progress check?

8. Are there any alternative or complementary therapies I can consider?

9. What are the warning signs that I should watch for regarding my condition?

10. Are there any dietary or exercise recommendations specific to my condition?

11. How can I manage any discomfort or pain associated with my condition?

12. Should I be concerned about potential interactions with other medications or supplements I am currently taking?

13. Are there any preventive measures I can take to reduce the risk of recurrence or complications?

14. When should I seek immediate medical attention or go to the emergency room?

15. Can you provide me with resources or additional information about my condition for further understanding?

Feel free to modify and add any specific questions based on your individual health situation to ensure that all your concerns are addressed during your visit.

When visiting an optometrist for an eye examination or for any specific eye-related concerns, it is important to ask relevant questions to ensure you fully understand your eye health and any recommended treatments. Here is a detailed list of questions you may consider asking your optometrist:

1. What is my current vision prescription, and do I need any corrective lenses?
2. Are there any changes in my vision that I should be aware of?

3. How often should I have my eyes examined for optimal eye health?

4. Are there any underlying eye conditions or diseases that I should be concerned about?

5. Do I have any risk factors for developing eye conditions such as glaucoma, cataracts, or macular degeneration?

6. Are there any measures I can take to protect my eyes from digital eye strain or other environmental factors?

7. Can you provide tips for maintaining good eye health and preventing eye problems in the future?

8. Are there any specific dietary recommendations or supplements that can benefit my eye health?

9. Should I be using any specific eye drops or treatments for dry eyes or other eye conditions?

10. Can you explain any test results or findings from my eye examination in detail?

11. Are there any recommended lifestyle changes or habits that can improve my overall eye health?

12. Are there any warning signs or symptoms that I should watch for that may indicate a serious eye condition?

13. What are the treatment options available for any diagnosed eye conditions and what are the potential risks or side effects?

14. Should I be concerned about any changes in my eye health as I age?

15. Are there any specific recommendations for protecting my eyes during outdoor activities or sports?

Feel free to add any specific questions related to your individual eye health concerns or any recent changes in your vision to ensure a comprehensive discussion with your optometrist.

As a writer and family woman, I believe that health tips are invaluable for the well-being of the entire family. By implementing healthy habits and lifestyle choices, families can significantly improve their overall health and quality of life. Encouraging good nutrition, regular exercise, proper sleep, and mental well-being not only benefits individuals but also creates a positive environment that promotes togetherness and happiness. Some helpful health tips for the whole family include:

1. Incorporate a variety of fruits and vegetables into meals for a balanced diet.

2. Engage in physical activities together such as family walks, bike rides, or sports games.

3. Limit screen time and encourage outdoor play or other activities that promote movement.

4. Make water the primary beverage choice and limit sugary drinks.

5. Plan and prepare meals together to teach children about healthy eating habits.

6. Prioritize regular sleep schedules and create a calming bedtime routine.

7. Practice mindfulness and stress-reduction techniques as a family, such as deep breathing exercises or meditation.

8. Schedule regular check-ups with healthcare providers to monitor health and address any concerns promptly.

No one in the family likes getting shots, but! Here is a detailed list of immunizations recommended for all ages in the family:

1. Influenza (Flu) Vaccine: Recommended annually for all family members, especially young children, older adults, pregnant women, and individuals with certain health conditions.

2. Tetanus, Diphtheria, and Pertussis (Tdap) Vaccine: Recommended for adolescents and adults every 10 years to protect against these serious bacterial infections.

3. Measles, Mumps, and Rubella (MMR) Vaccine: Recommended for children and adults who have not been vaccinated or need a booster to protect against these highly contagious viral infections.

4. Varicella (Chickenpox) Vaccine: Recommended for children and adults who have not had chickenpox or been vaccinated to prevent this viral infection.

5. Hepatitis B Vaccine: Recommended for all infants and unvaccinated adults to protect against this viral infection that affects the liver.

6. Human Papillomavirus (HPV) Vaccine: Recommended for adolescents and young adults to prevent certain types of HPV infections that can lead to cervical cancer and other cancers.

7. Pneumococcal Vaccines: Recommended for young children, adults 65 years and older, and individuals with certain health conditions to protect against pneumococcal disease.

8. Meningococcal Vaccines: Recommended for adolescents, college students, and individuals with certain health conditions to protect against meningococcal disease.

9. Hepatitis A Vaccine: Recommended for children and adults to protect against this viral infection that affects the liver.

10. Shingles (Herpes Zoster) Vaccine: Recommended for adults 50 years and older to prevent shingles, a painful rash caused by the chickenpox virus reactivating later in life.

By ensuring that all family members receive these recommended immunizations, you can help protect the health and well-being of your loved ones at every stage of life.

Natural Remedies for the Whole Family:

1. Honey and Lemon: A classic combination, a mixture of honey and lemon can help soothe sore throats and calm coughs. Simply mix a teaspoon of honey with some fresh lemon juice in a glass of warm water.

2. Ginger: Ginger has anti-inflammatory properties and can be used to alleviate nausea, motion sickness, and digestive issues. You can brew ginger tea or add grated ginger to your meals.

3. Garlic: Known for its immune-boosting properties, garlic can help fight off colds and flu. You can consume raw garlic or add it to your dishes for added flavor and health benefits.

4. Eucalyptus Oil: Eucalyptus oil is excellent for relieving nasal congestion and sinus pressure. You can add a few drops to a bowl of hot water and inhale the steam or diffuse it in a room.

5. Chamomile: Chamomile tea is a calming remedy that can help with anxiety, insomnia, and digestive issues. It is safe for both children and adults to drink before bedtime.

6. Echinacea: Echinacea is a popular herb known for its immune-boosting properties. It can help reduce the severity and duration of colds and infections. Echinacea supplements or teas are widely available.

7. Aloe Vera: Aloe vera gel can be used topically to soothe sunburns, minor cuts, and skin irritations. It has healing and anti-inflammatory properties that make it a versatile remedy for skin issues.

8. Peppermint Oil: Peppermint oil is known for its cooling and soothing effects. It can help relieve headaches, muscle aches, and digestive discomfort. Dilute a few drops of peppermint oil in a carrier oil before applying it to the skin.

9. Apple Cider Vinegar: Apple cider vinegar is a versatile remedy that can help with digestion, weight management, and. Dilute a tablespoon of apple cider vinegar in a glass of water and drink it before meals.

10. Turmeric: Turmeric contains curcumin, a powerful anti-inflammatory compound. It can help reduce pain and inflammation in conditions like arthritis. Tur can be added to curries, soups, or taken as a supplement.

Remember, it's always best to consult with a healthcare provider before trying any new natural remedies, especially if you have underlying health conditions or are pregnant or breastfeeding.

Herbal Tea Recommendations for the Whole Family:

1. Chamomile Tea: Chamomile tea is a gentle and calming herbal tea that is safe for all ages. It can help reduce stress, promote better sleep, and soothe digestive issues. Chamomile tea has a mild, slightly sweet flavor that is well-loved by both children and adults.

2. Peppermint Tea: Peppermint tea is refreshing and invigorating, making it a great choice for boosting energy and aiding digestion. It can also help relieve headaches and nausea. Peppermint tea has a cooling menthol flavor that is enjoyed by many.

3. Ginger Tea: Ginger tea is known for its warm and spicy flavor, as well as its digestive benefits. It can help alleviate nausea, indigestion, and motion sickness. Ginger tea is also a comforting remedy for colds and flu.

4. Lemon Balm Tea: Lemon balm tea has a light and citrusy flavor that is uplifting and calming. It can help reduce anxiety, improve mood, and promote relaxation. Lemon balm tea is a great choice for unwinding after a long day.

5. Echinacea Tea: Echinacea tea is a popular herbal remedy for boosting the immune system and fighting off colds and infections. It has a slightly bitter taste, so you may want to sweeten it with honey or lemon.

6. Lavender Tea: Lavender tea has a floral and soothing aroma that can help reduce stress and anxiety. It is also known for promoting restful sleep and calming the mind. Lavender tea is a lovely choice for winding down before bedtime.

7. Nettle Tea: Nettle tea is a nutrient-rich herbal tea that can support overall health and well-being. It is high in vitamins and minerals and may help with allergies, inflammation, and improving circulation. Nettle tea has a grassy and earthy flavor.

8. Hibiscus Tea: Hibiscus tea is a vibrant and tart herbal tea that is rich in antioxidants. It can help lower blood pressure, support heart health, and boost the immune system. Hibiscus tea is enjoyed both hot and cold.

Remember to consult with a healthcare provider before introducing new herbal teas into your family's routine, especially if you have any underlying health conditions or are pregnant or breastfeeding. Enjoy exploring the wonderful world of herbal teas and their many benefits!

Taking medications properly is crucial for managing health conditions and ensuring their effectiveness. Firstly, it is important to follow the prescribed dosage and schedule given by your healthcare provider. Make sure to read the instructions on the medication label carefully and understand how to take it correctly. Some medications need to be taken with food or water, while others should be taken on an empty stomach. It is important not to skip doses or double up on doses if you miss one. Use a pill organizer or set reminders on your phone to help you remember to take your medications on time. Be aware of any potential side effects and notify your healthcare provider if you experience any unusual symptoms. Finally, never share your medications with others or take medication prescribed for someone else.

Tips for taking medications effectively:

1. Follow the prescribed dosage and schedule.

2. Read the medication label instructions carefully.

3. Take medications with food or water if needed.

4. Do not skip doses or double up on doses.

5. Use pill organizers or set reminders to help you remember.

6. Be aware of potential side effects.

7. Notify your healthcare provider of any unusual symptoms.

8. Never share medications with others or take someone else's medication.

Vitamin D

Vitamin D is an essential nutrient that plays a key role in maintaining bone health, supporting immune function, and regulating mood. It is primarily obtained through sun exposure but can also be sourced from foods and supplements. When taking vitamin D supplements, it is important to follow the recommended dosage provided by your healthcare provider. Vitamin D supplements come in various forms, such as capsules, soft gels, and liquid drops, so select the form that is most convenient for you. It is recommended to take vitamin D supplements with a meal that contains healthy fats, as vitamin D is fat-soluble, and absorption is enhanced in the presence of fat. Keep in mind that vitamin D can interact with certain medications, so consult with your healthcare provider if you are taking other medications to avoid any potential interactions. Regularly monitor your vitamin D levels through blood tests to ensure that you are maintaining optimal levels. Remember that while vitamin D is important, it is still possible to have too much, so be cautious about excessive supplementation and seek guidance from a healthcare professional.

Here is a summary list of the ideal weight for men and children, along with some tips:

1. Ideal weight for men:

- The ideal weight for men varies depending on factors such as height, body composition, and muscle mass.

- A common way to determine a healthy weight range is by calculating body mass index (BMI).

- Generally, a BMI between 18.5 and 24.9 is considered healthy for most men.

- However, it's important to remember that individual body types and health factors should also be taken into consideration.

2. Ideal weight for children:

- The ideal weight for children also varies based on factors such as age, height, and growth patterns.

- Pediatricians often track a child's growth and development to determine if they are within a healthy weight range.

- It's essential for children to maintain a balanced diet, get regular physical activity, and have consistent medical check-ups to ensure they are growing and developing properly.

Tips for maintaining a healthy weight:

- Eat a balanced diet rich in fruits, vegetables, whole grains, lean proteins, and healthy fats.

- Limit the intake of sugary drinks, processed foods, and unhealthy snacks.

- Engage in regular physical activity, such as cardio, strength training, and flexibility exercises.

- Stay hydrated by drinking plenty of water throughout the day.

- Get an adequate amount of sleep each night to support overall health and well-being.

Remember, it's always best to consult with a healthcare provider or nutritionist for personalized guidance on achieving and maintaining a healthy weight.

What the BMI is and how to use it

Body Mass Index (BMI) is a commonly used method to estimate an individual's body fat based on their weight and height. It is a simple calculation that can help determine if a person is underweight, normal weight, overweight, or obese.

Here is how to calculate and interpret BMI:

1. Calculate BMI:

- BMI is calculated by dividing a person's weight in kilograms by their height in meters squared.

- The formula to calculate BMI is BMI = weight (kg) / [height (m)] ^2

- If your weight is in pounds and height is in inches, you can use the formula BMI = 703 x (weight in lbs.) / [height in inches]

2. Interpret BMI:

- A BMI below 18.5 is considered underweight.

- A BMI between 18.5 and 24.9 is considered a healthy weight.

- A BMI between 25 and 29.9 is considered overweight.

- A BMI of 30 or higher is considered obese.

It's important to note that BMI is a useful screening tool, but it does not directly measure body fat or consider factors such as muscle mass, bone density, or overall body composition. Therefore, it may not be accurate for every individual, especially athletes or individuals with a higher muscle mass.

It's always recommended to consult with a healthcare provider or a registered dietitian to get a comprehensive assessment of your health, including factors beyond BMI, and to develop a personalized plan for achieving and maintaining a healthy weight.

Encouraging tips for a family's healthy weight:

1. Meal Planning:

- Plan and prepare balanced meals together as a family.

- Include a variety of fruits, vegetables, whole grains, lean proteins, and healthy fats in your meals.

- Limit processed foods, sugary snacks, and excessive amounts of unhealthy fats.

2. Regular Physical Activity:

- Encourage family members to engage in physical activities together, such as walks, bike rides, or sports.

- Limit screen time and encourage outdoor play for children.

- Find activities that everyone enjoys making staying active a fun and shared experience.

3. Stay Hydrated:

- Drink plenty of water throughout the day to keep everyone hydrated and promote good overall health.

- Limit sugary drinks and opt for water as the main beverage choice.

4. Portion Control:

- Teach and practice portion control to help family members understand and maintain healthy eating habits.

- Use smaller plates and bowls to help control portion sizes and prevent overeating.

5. Set Realistic Goals:

- Set achievable and realistic goals for improving health and maintaining a healthy weight as a family.

- Celebrate and acknowledge progress to keep motivation high.

6. Encourage Open Communication:

- Create a supportive and open environment for discussing health and wellness goals within the family.

- Encourage sharing successes, challenges, and providing mutual support.

7. Lead by Example:

- Be a positive role model by prioritizing and demonstrating healthy habits for your family members to follow.

- Show enthusiasm and consistency in adopting healthy lifestyle choices.

Remember, fostering a healthy lifestyle as a family is a team effort and requires support, communication, and commitment from all members. Every small step towards a healthier lifestyle collectively contributes to achieving and maintaining a healthy weight for the entire family.

Here are six yoga poses that are safe and beneficial for people of all ages:

1. Mountain Pose (Tadasana): Stand tall with feet hip-width apart, arms by your sides, and palms facing forward. This pose helps improve posture, balance, and concentration.

2. Child's Pose (Balasana): Kneel on the floor, sit back on your heels, and reach your arms forward with palms on the ground. This relaxing pose stretches the back, hips, and thighs while promoting calmness.

3. Cat-Cow Pose (Marjaryasana-Bitilasana): Start on your hands and knees, alternating between arching your back upward (cat pose) and dropping your belly down (cow pose). This gentle flow helps to improve spinal flexibility and relieve back pain.

4. Downward-Facing Dog (Adho Mukha Svanasana): From a plank position, lift your hips up and back, forming an inverted V shape with your body. This pose stretches the hamstrings, calves, shoulders, and spine while building strength in the arms and legs.

5. Warrior II Pose (Virabhadrasana II): Step your right foot forward into a lunge, bending your right knee at a 90-degree angle while keeping your left leg straight behind you. Extend your arms out to the sides at shoulder height. This pose strengthens the legs, opens the hips, and improves balance.

6. Corpse Pose (Savasana): Lie flat on your back with arms by your sides, palms facing up. Close your eyes and focus on deep breathing and relaxation. Savasana promotes deep relaxation and helps reduce stress and anxiety.

These yoga poses are safe and effective for practitioners of all ages, providing a range of physical and mental benefits. Remember to listen to your body, breathe deeply, and modify the poses as needed to suit your individual needs and abilities.

Let's go family! Here is a family-friendly workout plan for general fitness that is safe for all ages. Each workout should take about 1 hour to complete, and you can do these workouts twice a week. You can change and rearrange the workout to fit each family member's capabilities.

Day 1: Full Body Workout

1. Warm-Up (5-10 minutes of light cardio and dynamic stretches)

2. Bodyweight Squats - 3 sets x 15 reps

3. Push-Ups - 3 sets x 10-12 reps

4. Reverse Lunges - 3 sets x 12 reps per leg

5. Plank - 3 sets x 30-60 seconds

6. Bodyweight Rows (using a resistance band) - 3 sets x 12 reps

7. Side Plank (both sides) - 3 sets x 30 seconds per side

8. Cool Down and Stretching

Day 2: Cardio and Core Workout

1. Warm-Up (5-10 minutes of light cardio and dynamic stretches)

2. Jumping Jacks - 3 sets x 30 seconds

3. Mountain Climbers - 3 sets x 30 seconds

4. Bicycle Crunches - 3 sets x 20 reps per side

5. High Knees - 3 sets x 30 seconds

6. Russian Twists - 3 sets x 20 reps

7. Burpees - 3 sets x 10 reps

8. Cool Down and Stretching

Exercise Modifications:

- Beginners or older adults can perform exercises at their own pace and intensity level.

- For individuals with mobility issues, low-impact options can be included, such as seated exercises or chair-assisted movements.

- Make sure to encourage everyone to listen to their bodies and not push themselves beyond their limits. Rest as needed and hydrate throughout the workout.

This workout plan focuses on overall fitness, incorporating strength, cardiovascular endurance, and core stability. It's important to have fun and stay active as a family while working towards your fitness goals. Remember to stay hydrated, wear comfortable clothing and supportive footwear, and enjoy the time spent exercising together!

4-day workout plan for your family focused on muscular hypertrophy. Each workout should take about 1 hour to complete.

Day 1: Upper Body Strength

1. Bench Press - 4 sets x 8-10 reps

2. Bent Over Rows - 4 sets x 8-10 reps

3. Shoulder Press - 3 sets x 8-12 reps

4. Pull-Ups or Lat Pulldowns - 3 sets x 8-12 reps

5. Bicep Curls - 3 sets x 10-12 reps

6. Triceps Dips or Skull Crushers - 3 sets x 10-12 reps

Day 2: Lower Body Strength

1. Squats - 4 sets x 8-10 reps

2. Deadlifts - 4 sets x 8-10 reps

3. Lunges - 3 sets x 10-12 reps per leg

4. Leg Press - 3 sets x 10-12 reps

5. Calf Raises - 3 sets x 15-20 reps

Day 3: Active Rest (Light Cardio or Yoga)

Engage in light cardio such as walking, cycling, or yoga to help with recovery and flexibility.

Day 4: Upper Body Hypertrophy

1. Incline Bench Press - 4 sets x 10-12 reps

2. Seated Rows - 4 sets x 10-12 reps

3. Lateral Raises - 3 sets x 12-15 reps

4. Face Pulls - 3 sets x 12-15 reps

5. Hammer Curls - 3 sets x 12-15 reps

6. Triceps Pushdowns - 3 sets x 12-15 reps

Day 5: Lower Body Hypertrophy

1. Leg Press - 4 sets x 10-12 reps

2. Romanian Deadlifts - 4 sets x 10-12 reps

3. Leg Extensions - 3 sets x 12-15 reps

4. Leg Curls - 3 sets x 12-15 reps

5. Standing Calf Raises - 3 sets x 15-20 reps

Day 6-7: Rest or Active Recovery

Take time to rest and recover or engage in light activities such as walking, stretching, or yoga.

Remember to progressively increase weight as you get stronger, and always focus on the proper form to prevent injuries. Make sure to stay hydrated, eat a balanced diet, and get enough sleep to support your muscle growth goals. Enjoy your workouts as a family!

A healthy sleep schedule and the environment!

I recognize the significant impact that a healthy sleep schedule and environment can have on families. I am passionate about exploring the importance of a healthy sleep schedule and environment. Establishing a consistent sleep routine for every family member is crucial for promoting harmony, well-being, and optimal functioning within the household. A well-rested family is more likely to experience improved communication, patience, and overall happiness. A consistent sleep routine is essential for overall well-being, as it allows the body to rest, repair, and recharge. Quality sleep has been linked to improved cognitive function, emotional well-being, and physical health. Creating a supportive sleep environment can enhance the quality of rest by minimizing disruptions such as noise, light, and uncomfortable temperatures. Creating a peaceful sleep environment for the entire family can also foster a sense of security and relaxation, leading to better sleep quality for everyone. Parents who prioritize a healthy sleep schedule for their children set a positive example and instill valuable habits that can benefit the entire family's physical and emotional health. By recognizing the importance of sleep-in family life and making it a priority, families can strengthen their bonds and support each other in leading healthy, fulfilling lives. By prioritizing a healthy sleep schedule and environment, individuals can optimize their daily performance, mood, and long-term health outcomes. It is easy to see that investing in healthy sleep habits is a fundamental aspect of self-care and deserves our attention and commitment.

In following this health information and maintaining a supportive environment that values wellness, families can cultivate a strong foundation for long-term health and happiness. Let's avoid the bags under the eyes, fatigue and rushed signs of early aging. Who wants that anyway right now? I thought not so get some rest at bedtime.

Key Takeaways: Men, Women, and Children's Health Tips

After exploring the chapter section on health tips for men, women, and children, here are the key takeaways to enhance overall well-being and promote a healthy lifestyle tailored to each demographic:

Men's Health Tips

1. Physical Fitness: Regular exercise, including cardio and strength training, is crucial for improving fitness levels and reducing the risk of chronic diseases.

2. Nutrition: A balanced diet rich in fruits, vegetables, whole grains, lean proteins, and healthy fats are essential for optimal health and well-being.

3. Regular Health Check-ups: Scheduling routine health check-ups helps monitor vital signs and address any health concerns early on.

4. Mental Health Awareness: Prioritizing mental health and seeking support for stress and anxiety is vital for overall well-being.

5. Avoiding Harmful Behaviors: Understanding the risks associated with smoking, excessive alcohol consumption, and other harmful behaviors is crucial for maintaining good health.

Women's Health Tips

1. Physical Activity: Engaging in regular exercise supports heart health, mood improvement, and overall well-being for women.

2. Healthy Eating Habits: A nutritious diet is essential to support hormonal balance and overall health for women of all ages.

3. Reproductive Health: Regular gynecological exams and breast health screenings are important components of women's health care.

4. Mental Well-being: Awareness of mental health and strategies for managing stress and anxiety are key for emotional wellness.

5. Self-Care Practices: Prioritizing self-care activities such as relaxation techniques and seeking social support can contribute to overall well-being.

Children's Health Tips

1. Healthy Eating Habits: Providing children with a balanced diet rich in essential nutrients supports their growth and development.

2. Regular Physical Activity: Encouraging children to engage in regular exercise promotes muscle and bone strength and overall well-being.

3. Routine Check-ups: Scheduling regular pediatric check-ups and following immunization schedules are important for maintaining children's health.

4. Limiting Screen Time: Setting limits on screen time and encouraging outdoor play and social interactions are beneficial for children's development.

5. Emotional Wellness: Supporting children's emotional well-being and providing resources for managing emotions help build resilience and promote overall health.

By integrating these key takeaways into daily routines and lifestyle choices, men, women, and children can take proactive steps towards improving their health and well-being at every stage of life.

Key Takeaways

Key Takeaway from "One Year Wellness Journey: The Family Edition":

The "One Year Wellness Journey for the Family" book is a valuable resource that focuses on promoting holistic well-being for the entire family unit over the course of a year. This book offers a comprehensive guide that addresses physical health, mental well-being, emotional balance, and spiritual fulfillment for each family member, with a particular emphasis on the interconnectedness of individual wellness within the family dynamic.

Throughout the book, readers are provided with practical strategies and actionable steps to foster a supportive and healthy family environment. The book highlights the importance of communication, cooperation, and mutual respect in cultivating strong family relationships and nurturing each family member's well-being. It encourages families to engage in activities together, practice gratitude, and create meaningful traditions that strengthen bonds and promote overall wellness.

Through following the guidance and suggestions outlined in "One Year Wellness Journey for the Family," families can expect to experience improved cohesion, enhanced communication, and a deeper sense of connection with one another. The book offers tools for implementing healthy habits, fostering positive habits, and creating a supportive network that empowers each family member to thrive and grow together.

Overall, the "One Year Wellness Journey for the Family" book serves as a roadmap for families seeking to prioritize wellness, create a harmonious home environment, and build lasting memories and experiences that contribute to a balanced and fulfilling family life.

Reflecting on a One-Year Wellness Journey and Celebrating Achievements

Author's Reflection

As the sun sets on yet another day, I find myself sitting in quiet contemplation, reflecting on the remarkable journey that the past year has been – a journey dedicated to my own wellness. It has been a transformative year, filled with challenges, triumphs, setbacks, and above all, growth. As I look back on how far I have come, I am filled with a sense of pride and gratitude for the changes I have made and the accomplishments I have achieved.

One year ago, I made a commitment to prioritize my well-being and embark on a journey towards a healthier, happier life. It was not an easy decision – it required dedication, discipline, and a willingness to confront my own habits and beliefs. I started by setting clear goals for myself, outlining the areas of my life that I wanted to improve – physically, mentally, emotionally, and spiritually.

In the realm of physical wellness, I made a conscious effort to adopt a more active lifestyle. I incorporated regular exercise into my routine, whether it be jogging in the crisp morning air, practicing yoga to center my mind and body, or lifting weights to build strength and resilience. I revamped my diet, opting for nourishing, wholesome foods over processed junk, and learned to listen to my body's signals of hunger and fullness.

On the mental and emotional front, I delved into practices of mindfulness and meditation, learning to quiet the incessant chatter of my mind and cultivate a sense of inner peace and tranquility. I sought out therapy to address deep-seated emotional wounds and develop healthier coping mechanisms for stress and anxiety. It was a journey of self-discovery and self-compassion, as I learned to embrace my flaws and vulnerabilities with gentleness and acceptance.

Spiritually, I explored different avenues of connection and meaning, whether it be through nature walks that rekindled my sense of wonder and awe, or through volunteering and acts of service that nurtured my sense of purpose and altruism. I delved into spiritual literature and wisdom traditions, seeking guidance and solace in the age-old questions of existence, and meaning.

As I reflect on the strides, I have made in each of these dimensions of wellness, I cannot help but feel a profound sense of achievement. I have lost weight and resilience and cultivated mental clarity and emotional resilience and deepened my sense of connection and purpose in the world. But beyond the tangible outcomes, I have also gained a newfound sense of self-awareness and empowerment – the knowledge that I am capable of effecting positive change in my life.

Today, as I celebrate the one-year mark of my wellness journey, I do so with a heart full of gratitude and a mind brimming with possibilities. I am grateful for the lessons learned, the challenges overcome, and the growth experienced. I am grateful for the support of loved ones who cheered me on and stood by me through thick and thin. And I am grateful for the opportunity to continue this journey of self-discovery and self-improvement, knowing that the road ahead may be long and winding, but ultimately rewarding.

In reflecting on my one-year wellness journey it fills me with a sense of accomplishment and joy. It is a testament to the power of perseverance, dedication, and self-love. And as I move forward into the next chapter of my life, I do so with renewed vigor and determination, committed to nurturing my well-being and living a life that is truly aligned with my values and aspirations. I encourage you and your family to embark on your own one-year wellness journey. It is most definitely a lifestyle changer with some awesome benefits for yourself and family resulting in a healthy family legacy.

Toni W.

Resources for Help

Mental health

1. National Alliance on Mental Illness (NAMI): NAMI provides support, education, and advocacy for individuals and families affected by mental health conditions, including resources specifically tailored for children and adolescents.

2. Child Mind Institute: This organization offers a range of resources and information related to children's mental health, including tips for parents, educational resources, and access to expert clinicians.

3. Substance Abuse and Mental Health Services Administration (SAMHSA): SAMHSA provides information and resources related to mental health and substance abuse, including a national helpline for individuals in need of support.

4. National Institute of Mental Health (NIMH): NIMH offers research-based information on mental health conditions, treatment options, and resources for children and adolescents experiencing mental health challenges.

5. The Trevor Project: This organization focuses on mental health and crisis intervention services for LGBTQ youth, offering a 24/7 crisis hotline and support resources.

6. American Academy of Child and Adolescent Psychiatry (AACAP): AACAP provides information and resources for parents, caregivers, and professionals on child and adolescent mental health issues, treatment options, and advocacy efforts.

7. National Child Traumatic Stress Network (NCTSN): NCTSN offers resources and support for children and families affected by

trauma, including information on trauma-informed care and evidence-based treatments.

These national resources can serve as valuable tools for parents, caregivers, and children in need of mental health support and guidance.

Physical health

1. Centers for Disease Control and Prevention (CDC): The CDC provides a wide range of information and resources on physical health topics such as nutrition, physical activity, vaccinations, and preventive health measures.

2. American Heart Association (AHA): The AHA offers resources and tools to help individuals maintain heart health, including information on healthy eating, physical activity, and managing risk factors for heart disease.

3. National Institutes of Health (NIH): The NIH offers a wealth of research-based information on various health topics, including resources on children's health, nutrition, exercise, and disease prevention.

4. Let's Move! Let's Move! is a comprehensive initiative launched by former First Lady Michelle Obama to promote healthy eating and physical activity for children and families, with resources and tools to support active lifestyles.

5. ChooseMyPlate: ChooseMyPlate is a nutrition education program by the USDA that provides resources on creating balanced, nutritious meals, portion sizes, and healthy eating habits for children and families.

6. American Academy of Pediatrics (AAP): The AAP offers resources and guidelines on pediatric health and wellness, including information on vaccines, healthy growth and development, and disease prevention.

7. National Institute on Aging (NIA): The NIA provides resources on healthy aging, exercise, nutrition, and preventive health measures for older adults to maintain physical health and well-being.

These national resources can serve as valuable tools for individuals and families looking to improve their physical health and well-being through education, guidance, and support.

Marriage Counseling

1. American Association for Marriage and Family Therapy (AAMFT): AAMFT provides resources to help individuals and couples find licensed marriage and family therapists in their area, as well as information on marriage counseling and therapy.

2. National Registry of Marriage Friendly Therapists: This resource helps individuals locate marriage therapists who specialize in working with couples to improve their relationships and address marital issues.

3. Psychology Today: Psychology Today offers a directory of licensed therapists, including marriage counselors, with profiles detailing their expertise and specialties, making it easier to find a suitable provider.

4. Gottman Institute: The Gottman Institute offers resources, workshops, and online tools based on research from Drs. John and Julie Gottman to help couples strengthen their relationships and improve communication.

5. American Psychological Association (APA): The APA provides information on finding psychologists and licensed therapists, including marriage counselors, as well as resources on relationship health and well-being.

6. National Association of Social Workers (NASW): NASW offers a directory of licensed social workers, including those specializing in marriage and family therapy, and provides resources on mental health and counseling services.

7. Good Therapy: Good Therapy provides a directory of licensed marriage counselors and therapists, as well as articles and resources on marriage counseling, relationships, and mental health.

8. Oak Cliff Bible Fellowship Counseling Center

OCBF Counseling Center is offering Telehealth Counseling Services for individuals, married couples, family, children, and youth. 7140 Library Lane

Dallas, TX 75232

https://www.ocbfchurch.org/ministries/counseling-center/counseling-forms/

These national resources can help individuals and couples find qualified marriage counselors and therapists to address relationship issues, improve communication, and strengthen their marriage.

General resources

1. Parenting workshops: Many local community centers, schools, and non-profit organizations offer parenting workshops on topics such as positive discipline, effective communication with children, and stress management for parents.

2. Family counseling services: Family counseling can provide support and guidance for families experiencing communication challenges, conflicts, or transitions such as divorce or blending families.

3. Parenting books and podcasts: There are many books and podcasts available that offer parenting advice, tips, and strategies for raising children of all ages.

4. Childcare and educational services: Local childcare centers, preschools, and after-school programs can provide parents with support and resources to help ensure their children's well-being and development.

5. Family support groups: Joining a family support group can connect parents with others facing similar challenges and provide a sense of community and understanding.

6. Mental health services: Access to mental health professionals, therapists, and counselors can help families navigate emotional and mental health issues that may arise within the family.

7. Financial assistance programs: Families in need of financial support can explore programs such as SNAP (Supplemental Nutrition Assistance Program), WIC (Women, Infants, and Children), and housing assistance programs.

8. Legal aid services: Families in need of legal assistance for issues such as custody arrangements, divorce proceedings, or immigration status can seek help from legal aid organizations.

9. Community resources: Local community centers, libraries, and churches often offer family-friendly programs and events that can provide opportunities for recreation, education, and social connection.

10. Online resources: There are many websites and online forums dedicated to providing parenting tips, resources, and support for families. Websites such as Parenting.com, HealthyChildren.org, and Parents.com offer articles, videos, and advice on a wide range of parenting topics.

1. National Parent Helpline: A toll-free helpline (1-855-4A PARENT) that provides emotional support and resources for parents and caregivers facing parenting challenges. Website: nationalparenthelpline.org

2. National Center for Missing and Exploited Children (NCMEC): NCMEC provides resources and support for families of missing children, as well as education and prevention programs related to child abduction and exploitation. Website: missingkids.org

3. Boys & Girls Clubs of America: A national organization that provides after-school programs, mentorship, and enrichment activities for children and teens in communities across the country. Website: bgca.org

4. National Alliance on Mental Illness (NAMI): NAMI offers support and education for individuals and families affected by mental health conditions, including resources for finding mental health care and navigating the mental health system. Website: nami.org

5. Feeding America: Feeding America is a national network of food banks that helps provide food assistance to families facing hunger and food insecurity. Families can locate a local food bank through the website: feedingamerica.org

6. National Domestic Violence Hotline: A confidential hotline (1-800-799-SAFE) that offers support, resources, and safety planning for individuals experiencing domestic violence and their families. Website: thehotline.org

7. Child Welfare Information Gateway: An information service of the U.S. Department of Health and Human Services that provides resources and information on child welfare, foster care, adoption, and family support services. Website: childwelfare.gov

8. Zero to Three: A national organization focused on promoting the health and development of infants and toddlers, offering resources and information for parents on early childhood development and parenting. Website: zerotothree.org

9. National PTA: The National Parent Teacher Association offers resources and support for parents, educators, and schools to promote family engagement in education and advocate for children's well-being. Website: pta.org

10. Family Promise: A national nonprofit organization that works to prevent and end family homelessness by providing shelter, support services, and resources to families in need. Website: familypromise.org

These national resources can help individuals and families find qualified help.

Conclusion:

As you reach the end of this one-year wellness journey book, I hope you are filled with a sense of pride, accomplishment, and renewed dedication to your well-being. Over the past year, you have embarked on a transformative journey of self-discovery, growth, and empowerment, and the progress you have made is truly commendable.

Throughout this book, you have explored various aspects of wellness - from physical fitness and nutrition to mental health and self-care practices. You have taken proactive steps to prioritize your health and happiness, and the positive changes you have implemented have undoubtedly impacted your life in meaningful ways.

As you reflect on the past year, remember to celebrate not only the milestones and successes, but also the challenges and obstacles you have overcome. Every setback is an opportunity for growth, every difficult moment a chance to learn and evolve. Your resilience, determination, and commitment to your well-being have shone through, guiding you through the ups and downs of this journey.

Looking ahead, know that wellness is a continuous process, a lifelong commitment to yourself and your health. Embrace the lessons learned, the habits formed, and the self-awareness gained during this year-long exploration. Carry forward the wisdom, strength, and inner resilience that you have cultivated along the way.

As you close this chapter and prepare to embark on the next stage of your wellness journey, remember that you are very capable of achieving great things, of living a life filled with vitality, purpose, and joy. Trust in yourself, be kind to yourself, and know that you have the power to create the life you desire.

May this book serve as a reminder of your progress, your potential, and the transformative impact of investing in your well-being. Embrace the journey ahead with courage, curiosity, and a deep sense of self-love. Here's to a future filled with health, happiness, and continued growth on your path to holistic well-being.

One Year Family Wellness Plan Worksheet:

Family Wellness Goals

1. Physical Wellness:

- Goal: Encourage regular physical activity for the whole family.

- Steps: Plan weekly family hikes or bike rides, enroll children in sports activities, schedule monthly check-ins for family challenges.

2. Emotional Wellness:

- Goal: Foster open communication and emotional support within the family.

- Actions: Schedule family meetings to discuss emotional concerns, practice active listening and empathy, plan monthly family fun nights to bond unwind.

3. Mental Wellness:

- Goal: Support each family member's mental health and well-being.

- Actions: Create a quiet space for individual relaxation and reflection, engage in family mindfulness exercises or meditation, encourage reading or creative activities.

4. Social Wellness:

- Goal: Strengthen family bonds and social connections.

- Actions: Plan regular family outings or game nights, host gatherings with extended family or friends, volunteer for a charitable cause.

Family Outings or Nights

5. Spiritual Wellness:

- Goal: Explore and nurture spiritual beliefs and practices within the family.

- Actions: Attend religious or spiritual services together, discuss values and beliefs during family meals, engage in gratitude practices or prayer sessions.

Family Progress Tracking

- Use a shared calendar or journal to track family activities, achievements, and goals.

- Set aside time for family check-ins to discuss progress, challenges, and adjustments needed.

- Encourage each family member to share their thoughts and feelings about the wellness plan regularly.

Sunday

Monday

Tuesday

Wednesday

Thursday

Friday

Saturday

Rewards and Celebrations

- Plan family rewards for achieving wellness milestones, such as a weekend getaway, movie night, or a special meal.

- Celebrate small victories and accomplishments as a family to reinforce positive behaviors and attitudes.

Family Wellness Notes

- Use this space to jot down any ideas, inspirations, or reflections related to the family wellness plan.

- Document any obstacles conflicts that arise and brainstorm solutions together as a family- Write down motivational quotes, affirmations, or reminders to keep the family motivated and engaged in their wellness journey.

"Family that exercises and eats healthy together, stays happy and strong together."

The One Year Wellness Journey

Family Well-Being Edition

Discover More

Non-Fiction

Daily Meditation

Daily Meditation is a way to reduce stress, bringing with it inner peace, and a healthy sense of perspective. Meditation is an experience, with daily practice sessions comes desired benefits. Mind and body practices focus on the interactions among the brain, mind, body, and behavior. As a result, the spirit is soothed maintaining the peace and harmony within your energy space. Improving mental poise, coping skills with illness, life's challenges and boosting overall health in addition to maintaining a sense of contentment combined with well-being. I will cover what meditation is, the benefits of practice, and lastly some of the popular types, yoga mudras, principles, and asanas, what chakras are, how to maintain their balance. In this book you will see how to meditate daily and its importance for a healthy and happy lifestyle. Included are some of my meditation scripts, tips accompanied by affirmations for you to try when you feel secure and ready.

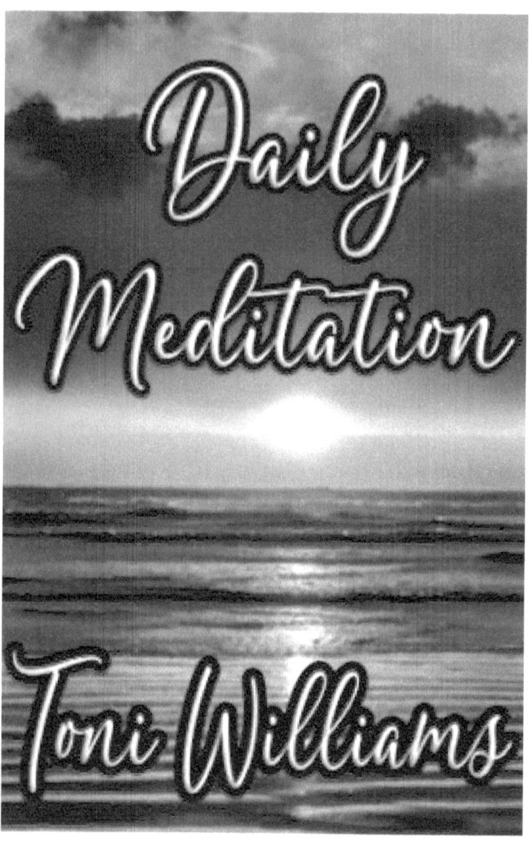

Daily
Meditation
Toni Williams

Young Adult Erotica Fiction

Hazel's Passion

Hazel Mackey is a red-hot, thick, and charming woman from Peaks. Her life is going nowhere until she meets herself for the first time in life. Hazel takes an instant indulging in her passion for running other people's lives in accord with her own personal prejudices. In her eye-opening experience, she becomes one of the most powerful and influential residents in the small mountain town of Peaks. Hazel also confessed to her share in the crime of passion, and the lovers eventually share her passion. Everyone that gets close to Hazel is easily aroused. Each caught in her web gives themselves to her fully and without remorse, despite knowing that their passion cannot last. Those that visit never want to leave and others have no clue about what this town really has to offer. A town well hidden, nestled and tucked away by mountains, old world style community. The best vacation spot to discover and unleash all your restrained passion. Visitors are encouraged to show pride, feel passion, and live the promise of membership. In pursuit of this passion all have put themselves through consuming passion that knows no limit, no boundaries. Peaks are warm, secretive, and an all-consuming fire when tempers flare.

No lawful passion can ever be so bewildering or ecstatic as an unlawful one.

Passion Forgotten Sparks

Four different unique stories of couples experiencing frustration, anger, and confusion. Something is happening to them all, unsure of what it is. The physical and emotional roller-coaster of sexual and relationship challenges they endure is only the beginning of an unexpected series of events. Leading the couples to meet themselves and or each other all over again; for the first time. Will they still feel as though their passion is restrained; or will some submit or even break? Over time many have forgotten to maintain the fire, which can result in dire consequences.

Hazel's Passion

Passion Forgotten Sparks

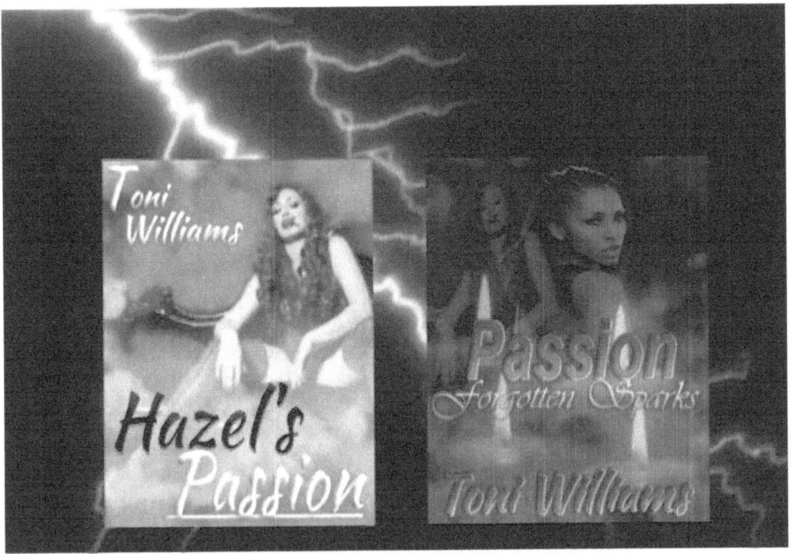

Poetry

Truth Syrum Series

https://www.smashwords.com/books/byseries/38962

- Truth Syrum Free to Speak

- Truth Syrum 2 Loud

- Truth Syrum 3 Spoken

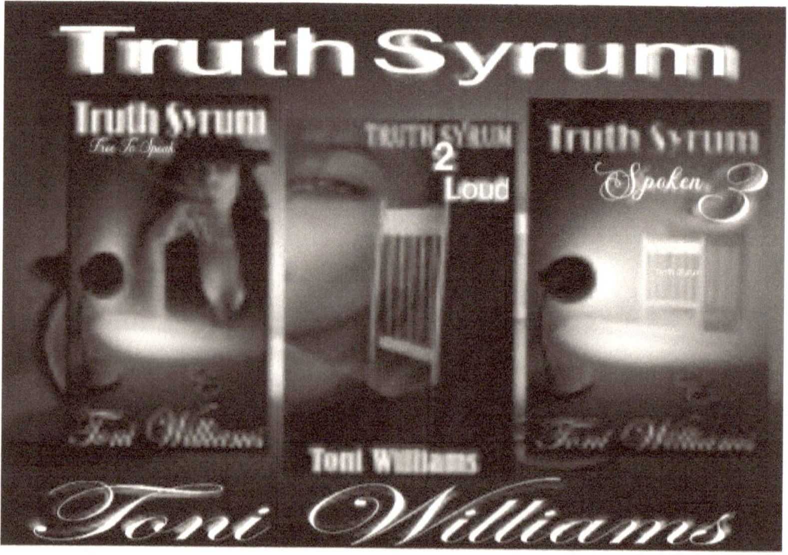

Truth Syrum Free to Speak

Free To Speak is the first book of the Truth Syrum series. A collection of poetry, interweaving the raw pain and pleasure of experiences. A young lady's battle in discovering the strength in learning, knowing, and speaking the truth. Life, tangled relationships, and deaths hanging in the balance, but something has and will happen as life goes on. Speaking up is neither easier said or done, especially when you are not free to speak.

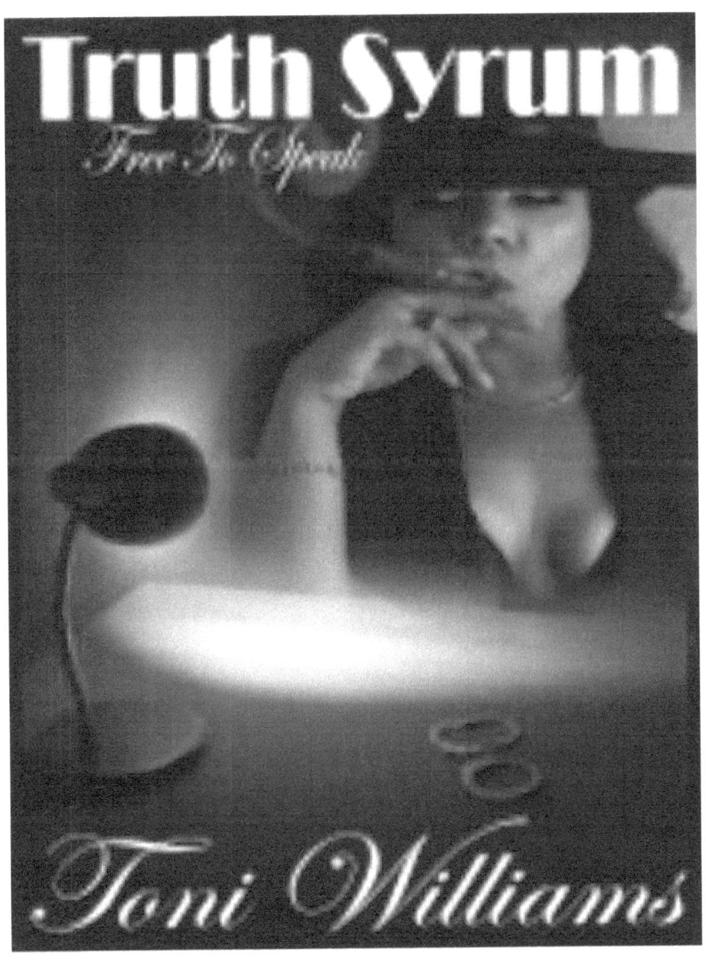

Truth Syrum 2 Loud

A collection of poetry, interweaving the raw pain and pleasure of experiences. A young lady's battle in discovering the strength in learning, knowing, and speaking the truth. Life, tangled relationships, and deaths hanging in the balance, but something has and will happen. It is inevitable; prepared or not, life changes without warning.

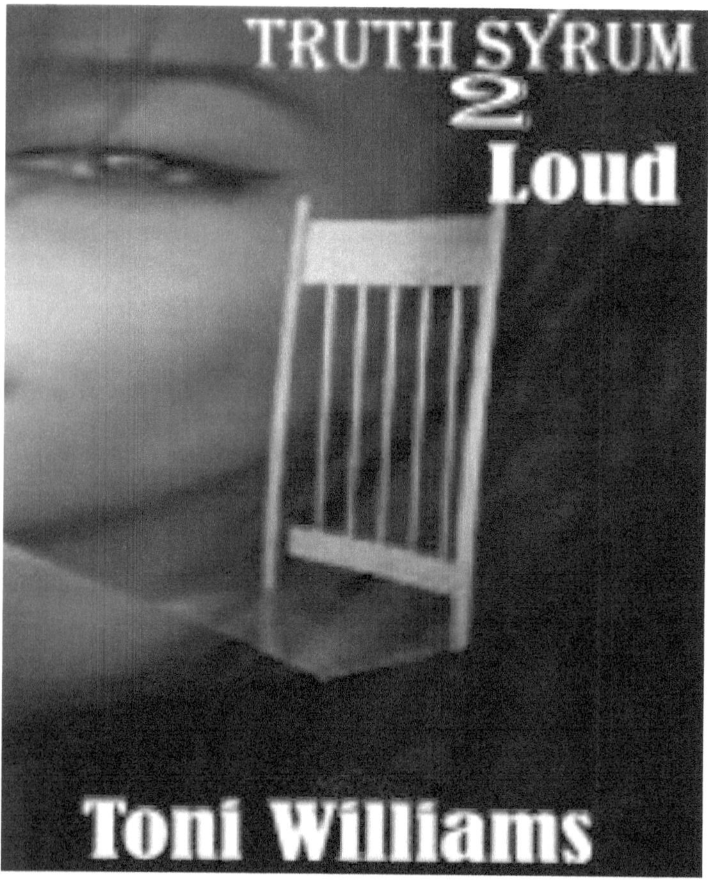

Truth Syrum 3 Spoken

Spoken is the third book of the Truth Syrum series. A collection of poetry, interweaving the raw pain and pleasure of experiences, a young lady's battle in speaking up. Now at the threshold of being heard, speaking out and attempting to get closure. Hoping to begin the healing process especially since she has finally spoken. Things take another unexpected turn, leading her down a new path.

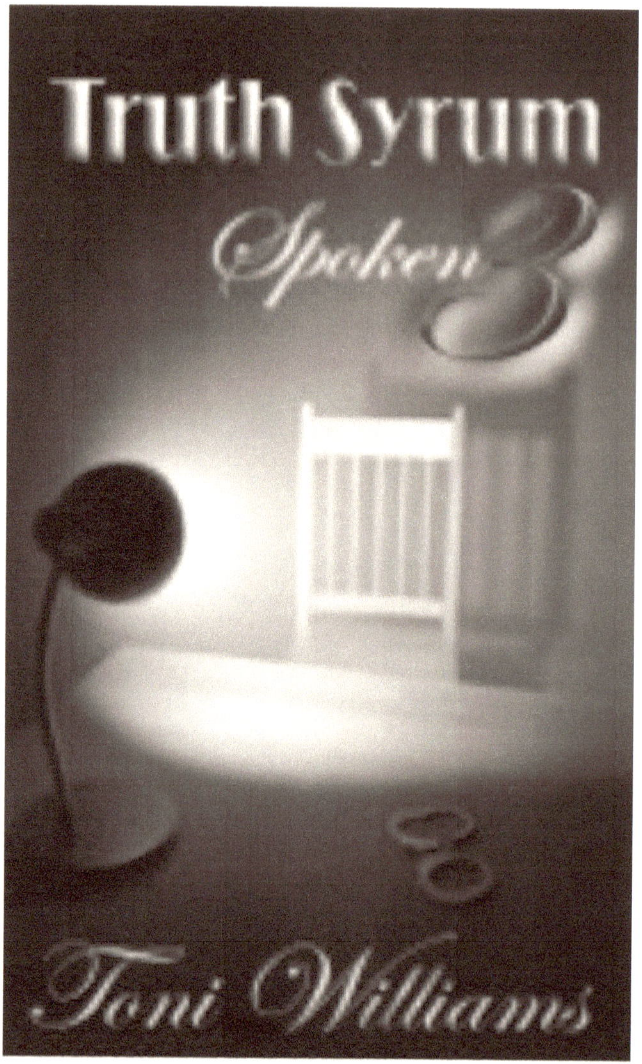
Truth Syrum
Spoken 3
Toni Williams

This book of poetry is some of the pains and pleasures of the heart. The heart endures battles on every end, day in and out, without a second thought. Taking on damage resulting in wounds and scars that may or may not heal properly or at all. The heart can be described in many ways, but it is something about her heart that make it simply undeniable. Life is carried, brought, and cared for as in all things she does. Loving, fighting for all that is good. Open minded, hardworking yet soft as silk. Appreciating the smallest pleasures to standing on faith in challenges. It is an honor for the person she chooses to understand, love, cherish, protect, and adore her heart. Charm of the fourth kind, she is kind and pleasant in all ways until she is not.

Her Heart

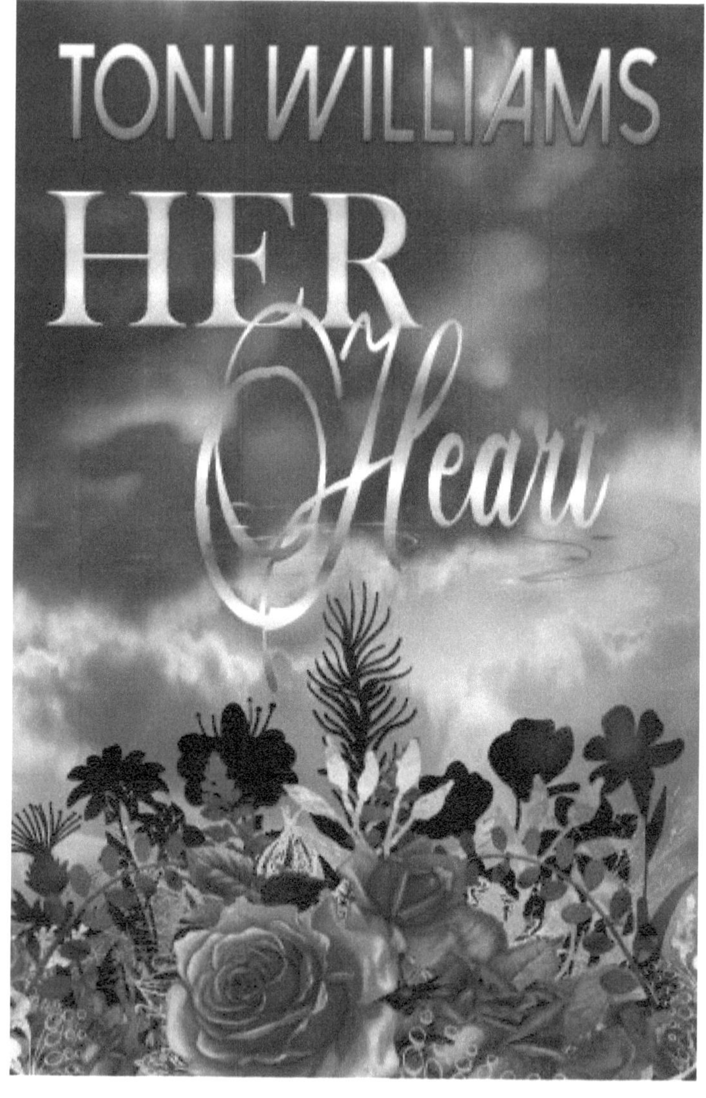

TONI WILLIAMS
HER
Heart

Children's Poetry

Words Early Poets

In this book we will learn unfamiliar words

and have fun playing with them. This book is a collection and introduction to poetry for young children. It is never too early for education and reading, to be an early poet. Reading is important, it starts with a word and then another and you are reading. With colorful and playful images young children can learn and have fun while learning.

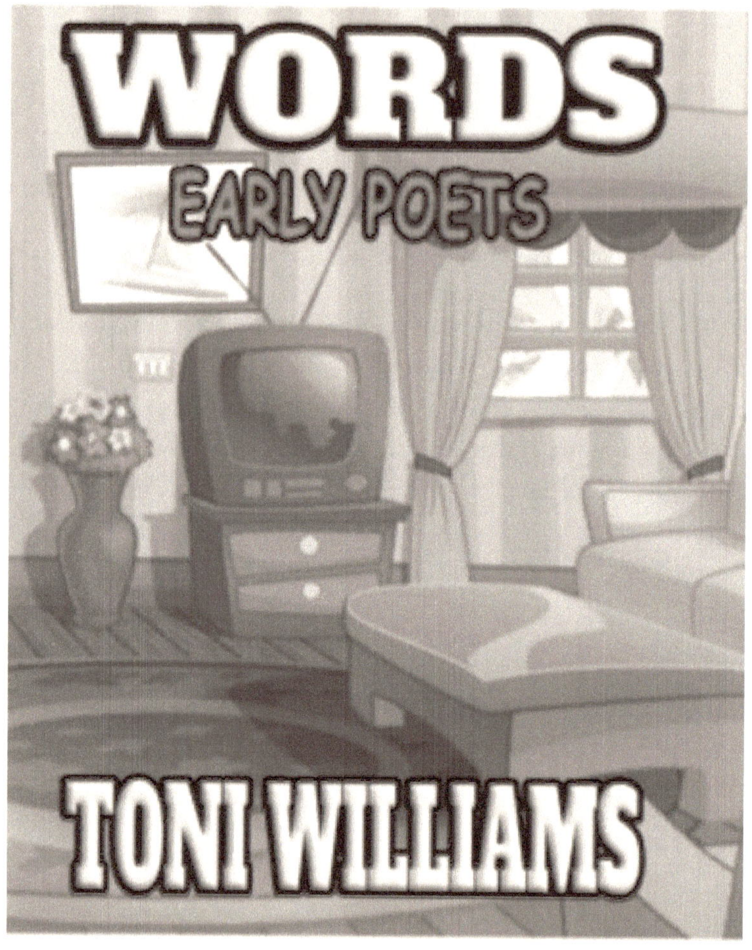
WORDS
EARLY POETS
TONI WILLIAMS

Children's Books

Words Early Poets

In this book we will learn unfamiliar words

and have fun playing with them. This book is a collection and introduction to poetry for young children. It is never too early for education and reading to be an early poet. Reading is important, it starts with a word and then another and you are reading. With colorful and playful images young children can learn and have fun while learning.

My ABC's Early Scholar

In this book we will learn the alphabet and unfamiliar words. Together we will have fun learning and playing with them. This book is an introduction to the fun world of education for young children. It is never too early for reading, to be an early scholar. Reading is important. It starts with a single alphabet.

Colors Early Scholar

In this book we will learn our colors and the differences. Together we will have fun learning and playing with them. This book is an introduction to the fun world of education for young children. It is never too early for reading and abstract art, to be an early scholar.

Reading, art, and creativity are important. It starts with a single alphabet, color, idea, and person. Education starts at home.

Numbers

In this book we will learn our numbers and how to count. Together we will have fun learning and playing with them. This book is an introduction to the fun world of education for young children. It is never too early for reading and math to be an early scholar. Reading and math are important, it starts with a single alphabet, number, and person; education starts at home.

Manners Early Scholars

In this book we will learn about our manners and when or where to use them. Together we will have fun learning and discovering manners together. This book is an introduction to the fun world of education for young children. It is never too early for reading and discovery, to be an early scholar. Reading and discovery are important, it shapes us into what we become. It starts with a single alphabet, child, and person.

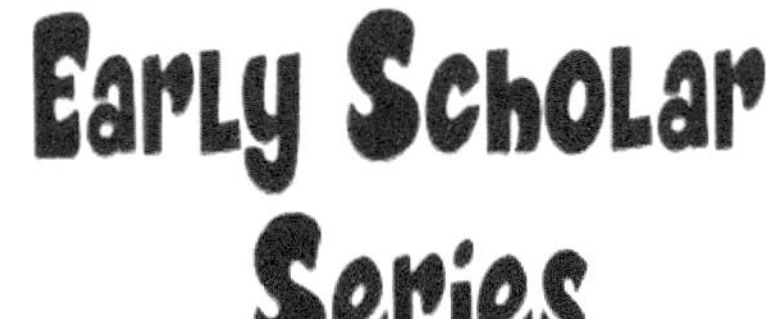

Early Scholar
Series

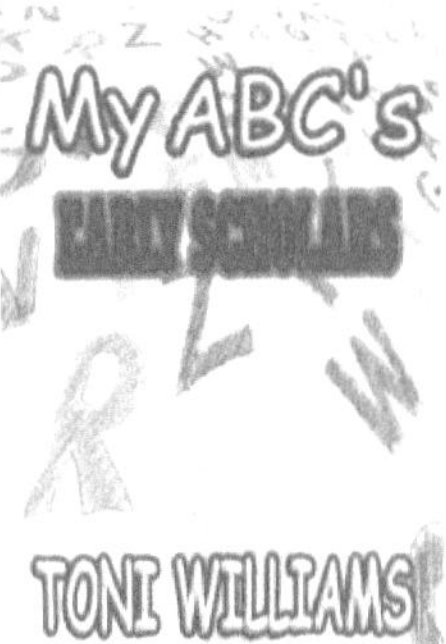

My ABC's
EARLY SCHOLARS
TONI WILLIAMS

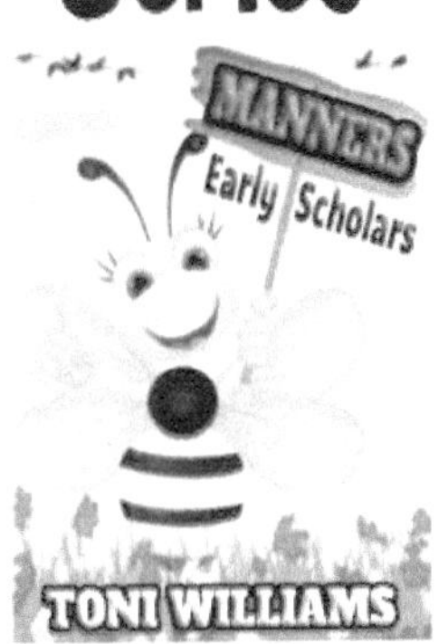

MANNERS
Early Scholars
TONI WILLIAMS

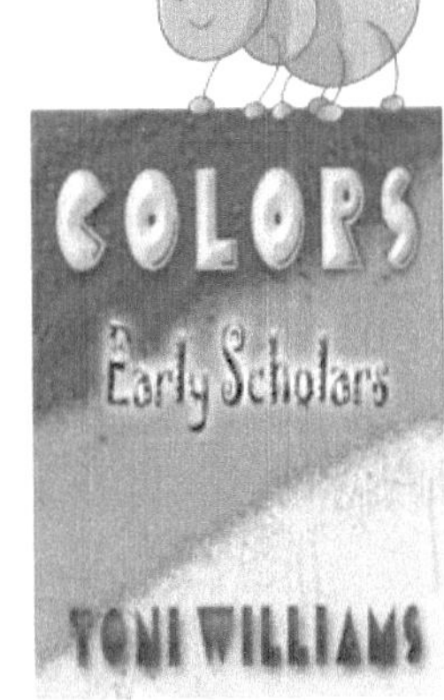

COLORS
Early Scholars
TONI WILLIAMS

Numbers

In this book we will learn our numbers and how to count. Together we will have fun learning and playing with them. This book is an introduction to the fun world of education for young children. It is never too early for reading and math to be an early scholar. Reading and math are important, it starts with a single alphabet, number, and person; education starts at home.

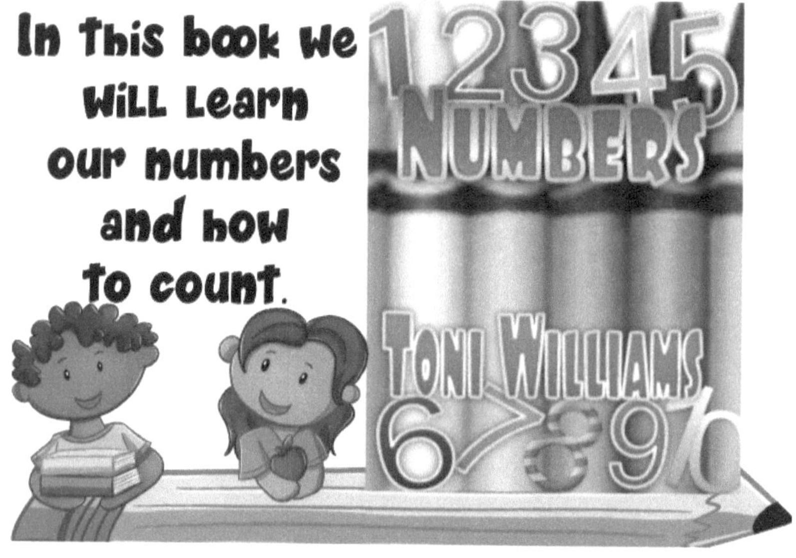

ABC's and 123's

We will go on an adventure learning the alphabet, numbers, colors, and some new words. Together we will have fun learning while playing with them. This book is an introduction to the fun world of education for young children. Early learning is great for building up memory, creativity, motor skills, confidence as well as a love for education. It is never too early for reading and to become an early scholar. Reading is important; it starts with a single alphabet.

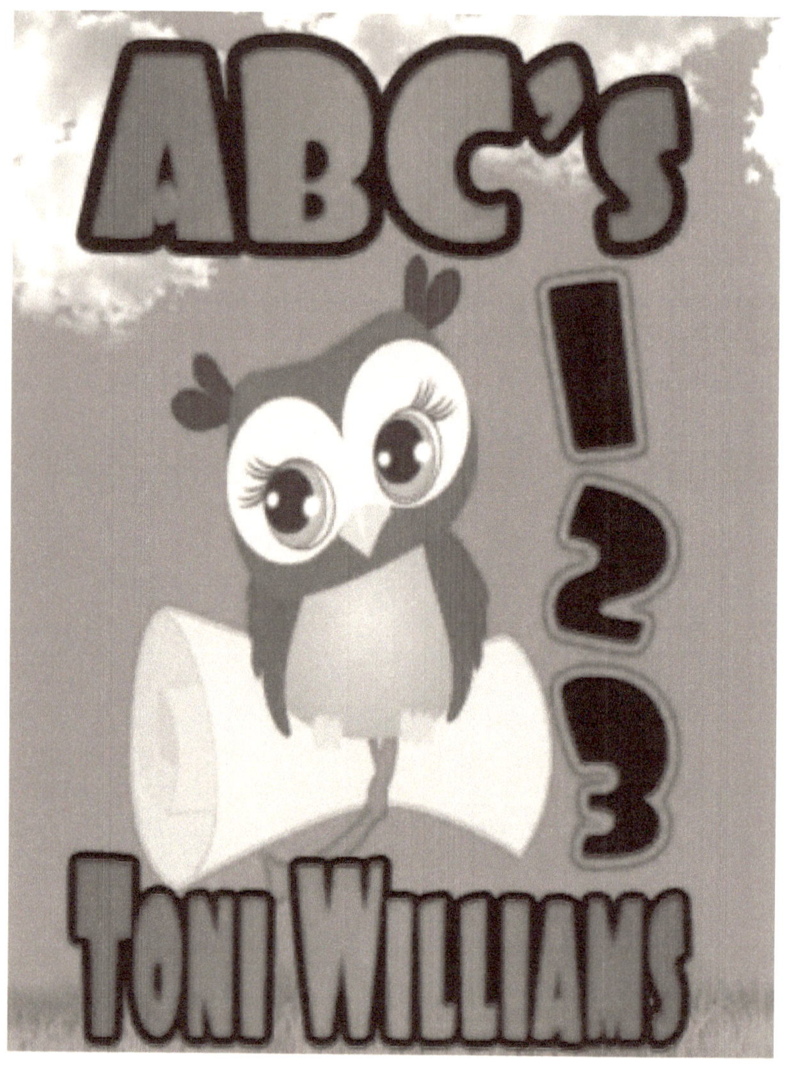

ABC'S
1
2
3
TONI WILLIAMS

Places we go

In this colorful book we will learn about our neighborhood and the places we go. Together we will have fun learning and discovering the many places we see and visit. This book is an introduction to the fun world of education for young children. It is never too early to be an early scholar. Reading and discovery are important, it starts with a single alphabet, place, and person.

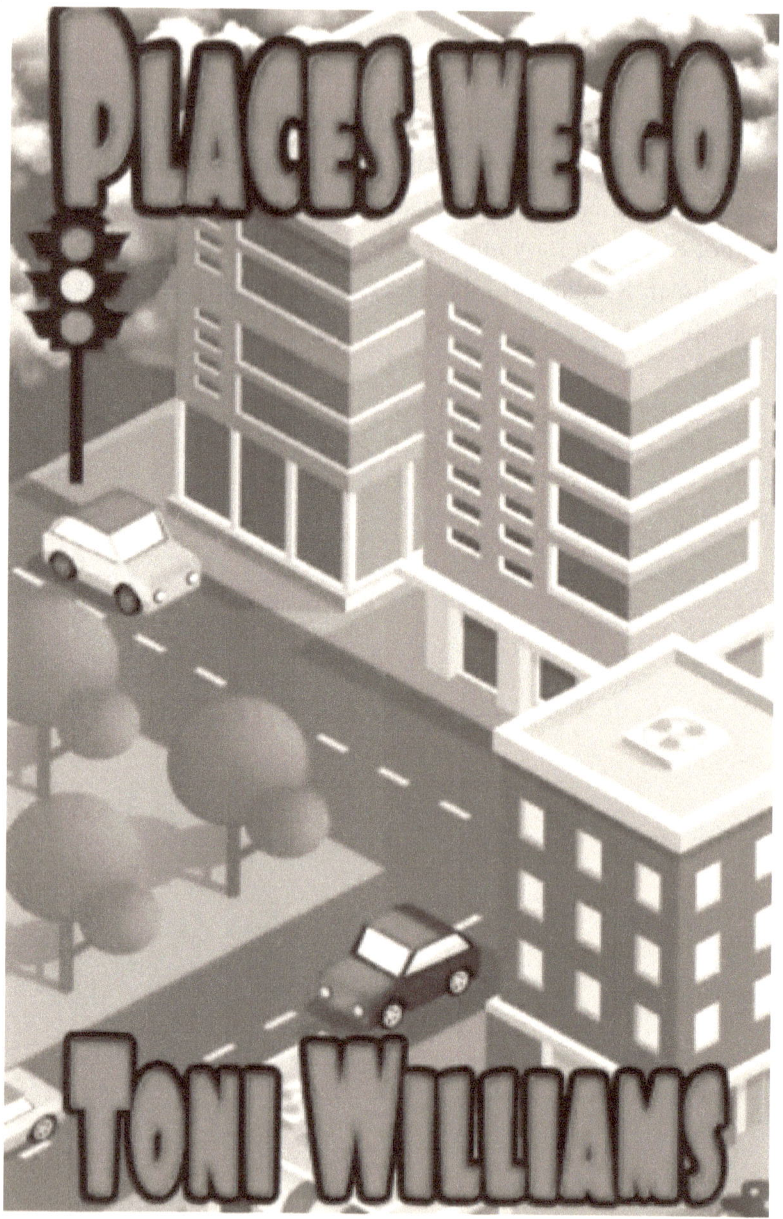

PLACES WE GO
TONI WILLIAMS

About Author

Toni Williams

I am a wife, mother, and grandmother who is also the owner and host of T On 1 Radio and its podcast shows as well as an author. I enjoy writing poetry, short stories to novels, erotica, mysteries, nonfiction, paranormal to fairytales, and children's books. Dedicated to, entertaining, uplifting, educating, and inspiring the world.

The experiences in life inspire me to reflect on my own life, problems, lessons, laughs and encourage me to tackle those challenges along with whatever life throws in along the way. Which in turn I share with the world to help others. Life is full of surprises with more inspiration to come.

Much love and respect to all-Toni

Thank you for taking some time to read my book.

If you enjoyed reading The Wellness Journey, please take a moment to leave me a review at your favorite retailer.

https://www.smashwords.com/profile/view/AuthorToniWilliams

Toni Williams

###

Don't miss out!

Visit the website below and you can sign up to receive emails whenever Toni Williams publishes a new book. There's no charge and no obligation.

https://books2read.com/r/B-A-VJRK-YIFBF

BOOKS2READ

Connecting independent readers to independent writers.

Did you love *One Year Wellness Journey*? Then you should read *Faith A Powerful Journey*[1] by Stephanie Christopher!

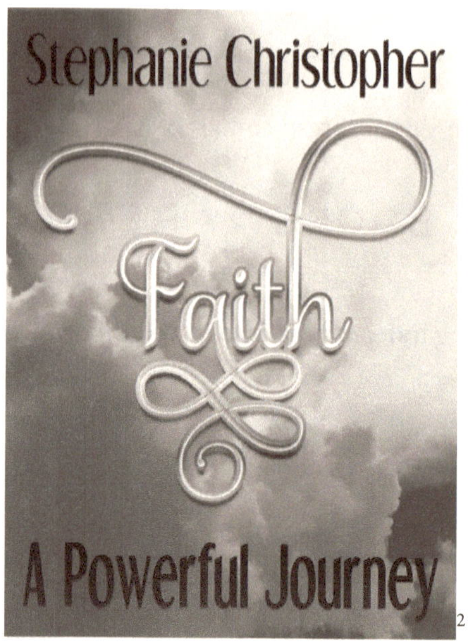

[2]

I extend to you a heartfelt invitation to embark on a powerful journey of faith through the immersive pages of my latest book, "Faith: A Powerful Journey." It is with great joy and anticipation that I share this invitation with you, as I believe in the transformative power that lies within the embrace of faith.

In "Faith: A Powerful Journey," I have striven to weave together a tapestry of stories, teachings, and personal reflections that will uplift your spirit, challenge your perspective, and ignite the flame of faith within your heart. This book is a testament to the extraordinary potential that lies within each and every one of us when we choose to surrender ourselves to faith's guiding light.

---

1. https://books2read.com/u/bx62L6

2. https://books2read.com/u/bx62L6

Allow me to guide you through the labyrinthine complexities of doubt and uncertainty and into the reassuring embrace of faith. Through the pages of this book, we'll explore the unshakable foundation of faith, the comforting solace it provides during life's trials, and the awe-inspiring miracles that can manifest through unwavering belief.

"Faith: A Powerful Journey" is not just a collection of words; it is a catalyst for personal transformation. Its pages offer a sanctuary for introspection and self-discovery, where you can find solace and guidance in times of doubt and a renewed sense of purpose when faced with adversity. As you delve further into its chapters, you'll find that faith is not a passive act but an active force that propels us towards a life of fulfillment and divine purpose.

Through my own experiences and those of others, I aim to provide you with the tools necessary to cultivate a stronger, unwavering faith in your own life. Together, we will explore the depths of belief, unlock the latent potential within you, and allow faith to guide you towards a life filled with purpose, joy, and divine guidance.

So, dear reader, I implore you to join me on this sacred journey. Let us embark on a path that connects us to something greater than ourselves, enabling us to transcend our limitations, and empowering us to live a life anchored in resolute faith. Open yourself up to the transformative power of "Faith: A Powerful Journey" and allow its message to resonate within the depths of your soul.

I eagerly await the privilege of accompanying you on this extraordinary voyage, where together we will unearth the boundless potential that awaits within the embrace of faith's profound mysteries

With abounding gratitude and unwavering faith, Stephanie Christopher.